Painting
the
Energy Body

Signs and Symbols for Vibrational Healing

Petra Neumayer and Roswitha Stark

Translated by Stephen E. Flowers

Healing Arts Press
Rochester, Vermont • Toronto, Canada

Healing Arts Press
One Park Street
Rochester, Vermont 05767
www.HealingArtsPress.com

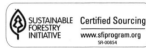

Text stock is SFI certified

Healing Arts Press is a division of Inner Traditions International

Originally Published in German under the title *Medizin zum Aufmalen: Heilen durch Informationsübertragung und Neue Homöopathie—Praxiserfahrungen mit den Körbler'schen Zeichen*
First U.S. edition published in 2013 by Healing Arts Press

Note to the reader: This book is intended as an informational guide. The remedies, approaches, and techniques described herein are meant to supplement, and not to be a substitute for, professional medical care or treatment. They should not be used to treat a serious ailment without prior consultation with a qualified health care professional.

Library of Congress Cataloging-in-Publication Data
Neumayer, Petra, 1960–
  [Medizin zum Aufmalen. English]
  Painting the energy body : signs and symbols for vibrational healing / Petra Neumayer and Roswitha Stark ; translated by Stephen E. Flowers. — First U.S. edition.
    p. cm.
  Summary: "Harnessing the power of symbols for physical, emotional, and spiritual healing" —Provided by publisher.
  Includes index.
  ISBN 978-1-59477-480-5 (pbk.) — ISBN 978-1-62055-145-5 (e-book)
  1. Energy medicine. 2. Vibration—Therapeutic use. 3. Signs and symbols—Psychological aspects.
  I. Stark, Roswitha, 1959– II. Title.
  RZ421.N4813 2013
  615.8'52—dc23
                                                                                            2012045196

Printed and bound in the United States by Lake Book Manufacturing, Inc.
The text stock is SFI certified. The Sustainable Forestry Initiative® program promotes sustainable forest management.

10 9 8 7 6 5 4 3 2 1

Text design and layout by Brian Boynton
This book was typeset in Garamond Premier Pro with Gill Sans used as the display typeface

Artwork by Alvina M. Kreipl, Kolbermoor; Petra Neumayer (pages 19, 122); Heike Brückner (pages 8, 12, 21, 26, 67, 84, 88, 94, 127, 134); BilderBox.com (pages 89, 105, 130); schwamedico GmbH (page 36); Koha-Verlag (page 68—Masaru Emoto)

Case studies by Renate Schertle ("Toothache," page 16), Christina Baumann ("Acute Injury," page 18; "Wound Healing," page 28), Felicitas Sperr ("Protection from Mosquitos," page 33; "Learning Difficulties," page 125), Roswitha Stark ("Tinnitus," page 71; "Disturbed Sleep," page 18; "Thyroid Nodules and Large Burn Scar on the Neck," page 91; "Chakra Treatment, page 120), Ursula Höll ("Atopic Eczema," page 97), Helga Bernardi ("Attention Deficit Disorder," page 99; "Bedwetting at Seven Years of Age," page 132), Angelika Dlouhy ("Sinusitis," page 102), Layena Bassols Rheinfelder ("Hay Fever," page 108; "Fear and Panic Attacks," page 113), Rudolf Fridum ("Animal Case Studies," pages 136–40); Regine Mühlhausen ("Treating an Oleander Plant," page 140).

To send correspondence to the author of this book, mail a first-class letter to the author c/o Inner Traditions • Bear & Company, One Park Street, Rochester, VT 05767, and we will forward the communication, or contact the authors directly at **www.medizin-zum-aufmalen .de/kontakt.html**.

Painting
the
Energy Body

Contents

Part I
Basic Knowledge

Part II
Practical Uses

Part III
Expanded Vibratory Balance

Preface

We recall the moment in 2005 when the idea for writing this book came about: Roswitha Stark and I had met during our training in practice-oriented homeopathy, and we were both immediately impressed by the inexhaustible possibilities offered by this gentle method of healing. Roswitha is a healing practitioner; in addition to her medicinal expertise, she brought excellent writing skills to this project thanks to her earlier career as an editor. I was trained in medical journalism, and the innermost impulse that drives me is the great question of what healing really is. It was destiny that brought the two of us together, so that we might join forces to show the world the revolutionary ideas of this new healing technique in our first collaborative book.

And yet, the search for a suitable publisher for this project was not as simple as we might at first have hoped. Try telling a publisher that you want to write a book about symbol medicine, let alone "painting the energy body"—make the sine curve symbol and the pain is gone! Hardly any publishers took our proposal seriously, or were willing to risk stepping into this unexplored terrain. But then, as luck would have it, we happened upon German publisher Raphael Mankau, who listened to our ideas with an open mind right from the beginning and, most importantly, had the courage to publish this first book on the topic! Now, thanks to Healing Arts Press, we have the opportunity to bring these teachings to the United States.

As freshly minted authors, we began with the term painting the energy body intending merely to broaden the horizons of homeopathy and provide our readers with a catchy, memorable term. At the time we had no idea what this would evolve into, that our ideas and our vision would lay the foundations of New Homeopathy through the introduction of new symbolic worlds.

Now, seven years since the publication of the first German edition of this book, we can take a moment to reflect on the experience. We are thankful that we had the opportunity to be "pioneers of words" and that our work has led to the establishment of New Homeopathy as an independent type of medicine for the well-being of humans, animals, and plants. Today, in the age of quantum science, informational medicine has an important role to play. Findings from the various areas of quantum physics are showing with increasing clarity that information (vibrations) are the building blocks and organizing force behind matter. The theories of Viennese electrical technician Erich Körbler (1936–1994), developed in the 1980s, are supported by the discoveries of epigenetics showing that our DNA functions somewhat like an antenna, sending and receiving vibrations. Thus, the sixty billion cells of the body communicate not only with one another but also with the outside world. As living beings, we are continually in communication with everything. And symbols, with their informational content, can be introduced into this plane of communication to send healing impulses into the organism.

The movement that has grown up around our work is so large that many other European therapists have begun using these methods, expanding upon them, and combining them with existing therapies. For doctors, healers, kinesiologists, and laypeople alike, the scope of healing with symbols seems to know no bounds—from the eye doctor who uses symbols to improve her clients' visual acuity to the healer who uses water transference to help children with ADHD escape Ritalin dependency. Likewise, we have been overjoyed by the praise, recognition, and thanks from the many animal healers and pet own-ers who have taken advantage of these methods to help the animals in their lives.

We would like to thank our instructor Layena Bassols Rheinfelder for her well-grounded teaching, which planted the seed that has sprouted so wonderfully in the past few years and is now putting forth fruit. We would also like to thank all the other teachers, colleagues, seminar participants, and friends who accompanied and supported us in this effort. Our heartfelt thanks also to the therapists who have enriched this volume by sharing their experiences with us in the case studies.

We wish you great joy and success in your application of New Homeopathy!

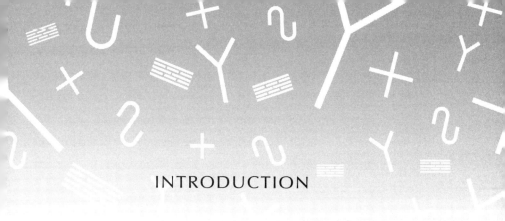

Healing Sickness through the Transmission of Information

The purpose of this book is to present a new system of energetic informational medicine, with all of its manifold possibilities. Whether you are a layperson, patient, or therapist, we hope this book will be informative and useful.

The name of this whole system of healing is New Homeopathy. It is based on the research of Erich Körbler, who rediscovered ancient knowledge and, through his own research, ultimately was able to bring together traditional Chinese medicine, the newest theories of quantum physics, and dowsing. He called this system of healing New Homeopathy because, like classical homeopathy, it is based on the idea of healing sickness through the transmission of information.

We are indebted to Körbler for making this knowledge available to a wider public, and for the fact that interest in this method of energy healing is steadily growing today. Many therapists have, in the meantime, built upon his knowledge, continued to research, to enrich New Homeopathy with their own experiences, or to link it to other supplemental systems of healing. From these additional developments have resulted a variety of names such as Practical New Homeopathy (PraNeoHom), Bioenergetic Regeneration Therapy, Sensory Resonance Therapy, and many more.

THE CORRECT VIBRATION
DOES THE TRICK

The theoretical foundations of the different methods of energy information medicine are all the same: everything vibrates. Stones, colors, microorganisms, people, geometric figures, etc.—everything that exists has a vibration, projects information, and communicates with everything else. If we equate a sick person with a musical instrument that is out of tune, then the organism could be properly retuned with the correct vibration. This is more or less the theory behind the many healing methods that heal with information and vibrations. They all have as their goal the harmonizing of a diseased organism by means of things such as colors, tones, frequencies, or symbols. When the harmonic "chord" within our resonant body is struck, energy flows again, and the organism receives new strength to allow the powers of self-healing to prevail. In this way illnesses are dissolved.

New Homeopathy is also based on this principle. It alters disharmonious vibrations with the help of geometric signs, according to the theory that every painted line functions like an antenna and alters the existing vibration. If these biophysically active signs are drawn on acupuncture points, for example, they painlessly stimulate the powers of self-healing. We call this practice "painting the energy body."

It is widely known that for thousands of years needles were used on the acupuncture points. Today, many different "meridian therapies" influence the meridian system and acupuncture points in varied ways, for example, by means of percussion (EFT), stroking, crystal acupuncture, the application of tuning forks, and so on. The painting of geometric signs on the acupuncture points can easily be viewed within this framework. It seems probable that the body painting of ancient peoples outside of the Chinese tradition—among American Indians, for instance, or the people who tattooed the famous ancient iceman, Ötzi—was similarly intended to bring vibrations into balance and engender healing.

Photos taken with an infrared camera by the Institute for Biophysics in Neuss, Germany, impressively show the circulation of different meridians. These images confirm that the meridian system is no invention of ancient Chinese dynasties, and suggest that it will soon be scientifically verifiable even to those who are skeptical of the Eastern therapeutic methods.

In addition to their application to acupuncture points, geometric signs can also be used for the production of informed healing water. The transmission of information into water is a very simple, effective, and low-cost technique that will be explained in this book: by drinking informed water it is possible to inform every cell in our bodies in a positive way.

New Homeopathy—and the methods and practices that have recently emerged from it—is suited not only to healing professionals but also to laypeople. These practices make it possible for every individual to care for his or her own health in a responsible manner—even in urgent cases. We can alleviate the pain of a swollen insect sting, for example, by drawing a healing symbol on the skin with a felt-tipped marker.

What is especially fascinating about this medicine is the

combination of its simplicity with the enormous bandwidth of its possibilities. By directly involving the patient, New Homeopathy promotes each person's responsibility for his own health and simultaneously imparts joy to this responsibility, which is independent and follows the laws of the universe.

Resonance therapies are understood holistically: the whole person (or animal or plant) is treated on all levels of being—body, soul, and spirit. For this reason a patient's relationship to her environment, living circumstances (social integration, familial and professional circumstances), psychological factors, radiation pollution (geological radiation and electrosmog), allergies, and environmental toxins all play a large role in our healing work.

REDISCOVERY OF INFORMATIONAL MEDICINE IN THE INFORMATION AGE

Erich Körbler dedicated his life's work to the meticulous research and recording of the system underlying vibrational medicine. He saw himself as a pioneer, while the colleagues who worked with him considered him a genius: a genius who especially distinguished himself through his creativity. In addition to Körbler's scientific work, which was honored with numerous prizes and awards, he was also interested in the arts and received a prize in Venice as a writer. The Belgian king awarded him a service cross, and EUREKA, the Center of the European Community of Innovative Research in Brussels, awarded him the gold medal.

Perhaps the most important creative work this joyous and unassuming man left to posterity is his New Homeopathy. The foundation of his healing system is the recognition that the human being is an informational system and can therefore be healed through information. Körbler's vision was one of a distant future in which people could be healed without chemical drugs and without invasive technical procedures—exclusively by means of informational transmissions. We are certain of one thing: the future has already begun!

We hope that the many practical examples and reports in this book will convince you of the same thing, and help you to realize that nothing is impossible! Come along on the journey and read how you can positively change your health with simple healing symbols.

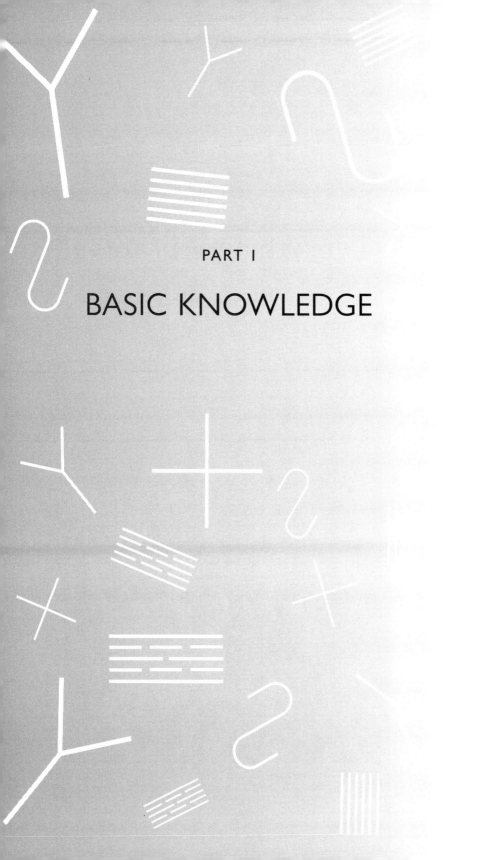

PART I

BASIC KNOWLEDGE

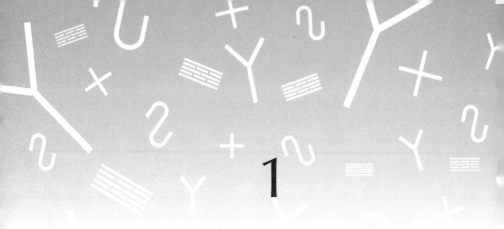

1

Everything Vibrates

Morphic Fields and Resonance

Whether animal, vegetable, mineral, or human, everything that exists vibrates and thereby constantly projects information. We exist in an open system in which everything is constantly connected to everything else. Two powerful principles articulate this worldview: the principle of morphic fields and the principle of resonance.

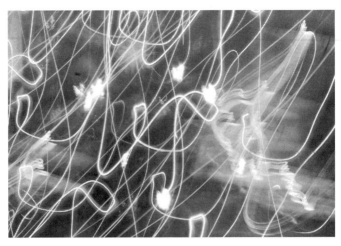

Light is a visual vibration.

Classical science assumes that developments in nature are guided by accidental processes and that we can come to understand the universe by dividing it into ever smaller parts. The English biologist Rupert Sheldrake looked at the world differently, however: in his research he turned to the question of how complex systems organize themselves. He suggested that we cannot get to know the painter of a picture by analyzing the colors in his painting. We can, however, conceive of the underlying thought, concept, or idea of this picture if we study the Whole. To begin to understand this concept of wholism, Rupert Sheldrake developed the theory of morphic fields.

MORPHIC FIELDS

Whereas mainstream science recognizes gravitational fields and electromagnetic fields, Rupert Sheldrake added theories of morphic fields. A morphic field is a field that provides form and organization. What makes single trees into a forest? Is it the arrangement between the trees or does a general concept lie behind it? Sheldrake held to the opinion that a wholeness—something like the organism "forest"—is organized by a morphic field, for the whole is greater than the sum of its parts. Every organized entity corresponds to such a field. The blueprint, the organizing principle, can also be called the collective memory of nature. Its form of expression is vibration—the equivalent vibration of similar forms over time and space.

A constant interaction exists between the morphic field and any organism: information is continuously exchanged. Even our own ideas, conceptions, and emotions generate a field. If we alter our thoughts and feelings, the field is modified in a corresponding way. Therefore we can say that we create our reality: we are the architects of our own destiny.

THE RESONANCE PRINCIPLE

Throughout our lives we are in constant communication and inter-action with our environment. Uncountable bits of information—vibrations—influence us from the outside and also radiate outward from our organism.

The concept of resonance originated in the work of the Russian biologist Alexander Gurwitsch (1874–1954). In addition to other important contributions, Gurwitsch theorized that everything vibrates and everything radiates. We can think of our own DNA as a type of "hollow space resonator" in the nucleus of each of our cells—similar to an antenna and transmitter.

Sometimes we can even feel such vibrations. When we meet a person we enter into a resonant state with him: we know in a fraction of a second whether we like him or not, whether he is on our same wavelength, or whether he "rubs us the wrong way."

If there is a vibrating tuning fork on a table, a non-vibrating tuning fork placed next to it will begin to vibrate: it enters into a resonance at the frequency of the vibrating tuning fork and operates as an antenna and transmitter at the same time.

It works the very same way with all vibrations that the human system encounters. We enter into resonance with the waves around us. The particular information that is transmitted to us by the waves we encounter often directs how our organism reacts: either the vibrations are wholesome for us, or they are unwholesome. The tolerance tests used by resonance therapies are based on this principle.

If, for example, we are confronted by artificially produced electrical or magnetic fields that make us feel unwell, then we call that electrosmog—that is, an unwholesomeness of these vibrations. Positive vibrations, on the other hand, act upon our organism in a harmonious way and can strengthen and activate the powers of self-healing.

In the figure below, the upper wave (the tree) has the same frequency as the vibration transmitted by the woman, though at a greater amplitude. This vibration is very well tolerated and strengthens the woman's own vibration. The greater amplitude does not disturb the wholesomeness.

If, however, two waves have differing frequencies, they can create an unwholesome disharmony that weakens our own vibration. This is made clear by the lower wave in the illustration. The vibration of the cat virtually clashes with the vibration of the woman, which is indicative of an unwholesome state.

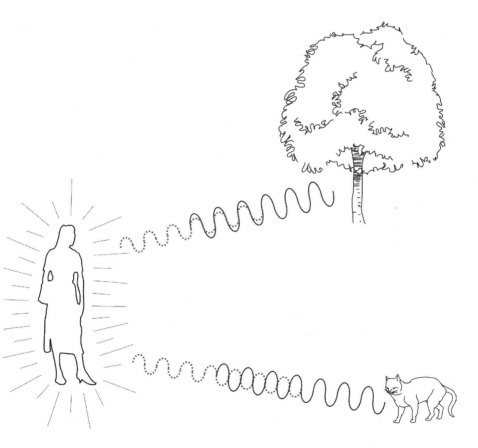

Our body's vibrations may be in harmony or disharmony with the vibrations of other organisms around us.

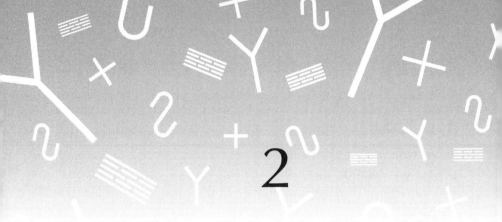

2

Healing with Geometric
Signs and Symbols

Geometric signs also transmit vibrations. If symbols are painted on the skin, for example, they can alter the vibrations in the energy field of the person or the flow of energy within him. The exact kind of change the symbols create will vary according to the placement and type of sign involved. This finding is the basis of so-called informational medicine.

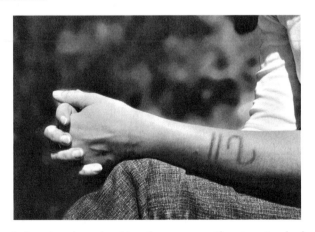

Symbols painted on the skin alter energy vibrations in the body.

The use of geometric signs and symbols to alter energy vibrations is no invention of modern times. Symbols have played a big role in all cultures, as they are the transmitters of energetic messages in condensed form. Body illustrations have been used all around the globe, from the South Seas to Africa to India and the Americas. In spite of divisions of time and space and without the possibility of contact between the different peoples, many cultures made use of similar geometric forms—for example, several parallel lines. A powerful example of this kind of body symbology was unearthed with the discovery of Ötzi, a 5,000-year-old glacier mummy, whose history of injuries was tattooed in lines and crosses on his body (see box on page 14).

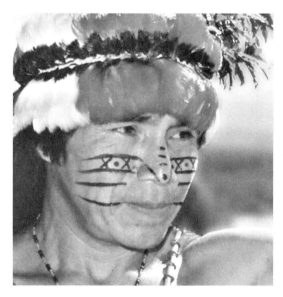

The lines and crosses shown here are symbols used around the world.

Some people react negatively to the idea of work with geometric symbols. This rejection occurs most frequently in European latitudes, where clergy in the Middle Ages tried to eliminate most traditions by means of Inquisition and witch trials, thus depriving the whole civilization of direct sensory experience with symbols for close to 500 years.

Is Ötzi Evidence for Acupuncture?

Ötzi was a corpse found frozen in the Tyrolean Alps in 1991; he was estimated to be at least 5,000 years old. Ötzi's body was tattooed with multiple lines and crosses; later research suggested that these tattoos marked the places where Ötzi was being "treated" for back and abdominal pain.

In a special conservation chamber, the fifty-seven linear tattoos were measured and photographed and then compared with the acupuncture points of traditional Chinese medicine (TCM). The results were astounding: most of the points correlated with the classical points of acupuncture, and many were on the Bladder meridian. From this the meridian therapy experts examining Ötzi speculated that the arthritis in his lumbar vertebrae and leg joints was being treated by these symbols. Linear tattoos on his Gall Bladder, Liver, and Spleen meridians suggested that he also suffered from gastrointestinal disorders. In any case these results open the door for new discussions as to whether acupuncture really had its origin in China or perhaps farther to the west in Eurasia.

Independent of acupuncture, there are also other teachings and systems concerned with circulation of energy and points of energy in the body, such as the trigger points according to Janet Simons and Peter Travell and the Head zones or points used in Japanese Reiki. From yoga and tantra we know about the energy rivers called "nadis"—ancient Indian writings discuss between 77,000 and 350,000 of these pathways in the body.

Healing with geometric signs has nothing to do with sorcery or magic; instead, it is a matter of rediscovering the long-lost knowledge of our ancestors, which is returning to us from many directions. Great thinkers in fields as diverse as physics, biology, and psychology have explored the power of symbols in recent times, from physicists studying quantum mechanics to Carl Jung, whose theory of the collective unconscious showed that symbolic material in the morphic field is stored in archetypal figures and mandalas.

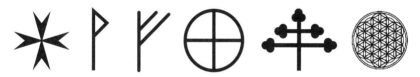

Symbols are omnipresent: Maltese cross, Wunjo rune, Fehu rune, wheel cross, Cardinal cross, Flower of Life

HEALING SYMBOLS

A healing symbol (from the Greek *symbolon,* meaning "connection") is a visible sign whose connective power can effect a wholesome vibration between that which provides the form (sickness, pain) and the ideal state—that is, between matter and consciousness. It was Erich Körbler who rediscovered an underlying pattern behind the most common symbols in the world. He identified these common elements: one to nine parallel lines, the equilateral cross that can be constructed from these lines, the Ypsilon/Life rune, and the sine curve.

All of the symbols or geometric signs shown on the following pages were developed from these simple forms or their combinations. In the following sections you will learn how New Homeopathy works with these signs and how you can discover what sign should be used in which case by using the single-handed divining rod or tensor.

SINE CURVE
THE SYMBOL OF REVERSAL

The sine curve is always a symbol of change or reversal. It transforms unwholesome information into wholesome—and the reverse as well; therefore this sign should be used with care. For example, if this sign is used too long, the positive is reversed back to the negative.

The sine curve can be painted directly on the skin and can also be independently employed to redirect all sorts of unwholesome information (disorders, illnesses, negative beliefs, etc.).

CASE STUDY

Toothache

A female friend of mine had been having a light toothache off and on for a few days. It was Christmas and I had been invited to her place for dinner. When I arrived she had already prepared the food, but could not eat anything because of her toothache. I did not have my tools with me, so I simply drew a large sine curve on the cheek where the affected tooth was. Within a few minutes the pain had almost entirely subsided. My friend could enjoy her meal, we had a nice Christmas evening, and she was able to delay her visit to the dentist until after the holidays—all because of the healing sign on her cheek.

THE LIFE RUNE, YPSILON
STRENGTHENING

In contrast to the sine curve, the Y always works in a positive way: it transforms unwholesome information into wholesome information.

Information that is already wholesome—like a positive affirmation—is further strengthened by this symbol.

The Ypsilon is always used at the end of the chain in a successful water transmission to stabilize the information in the body in a permanent way. It is only seldom used on the body itself, and only for certain complaints.

The Ypsilon is a powerful form in the natural world. Antibodies have an Ypsilon form, and when they bind with cells they render bacteria or viruses harmless. If a tree grows in a geopathic zone of disturbance, the trunk will divide itself in order to evade any geopathic effect—virtually assuming an Ypsilon form. The water molecule is also Ypsilon shaped.

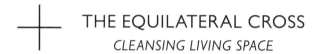

THE EQUILATERAL CROSS
CLEANSING LIVING SPACE

Although the cross is now known around the world as a Christian symbol, it was used in many ancient cultures. Note that it is only the equilateral, primitive Christian cross-form that works in an energetically positive and shielding manner: the Passion Cross that is created by shifting the horizontal beam upward has different energies. The protective character of the equilateral cross has even been noticed by real estate insurers in Switzerland, who have observed that houses whose windows are decorated with equilateral crosses have less chance of being burglarized.

In informational medicine, the equilateral cross mainly finds use in the cleansing of living space—for example, to free water veins or geopathic zones from interference. It has a protective effect rather than a transformative one; unwholesome radiation may still be present, but the body no longer reacts negatively to it.

The equilateral cross is seldom painted on the body, although some have found that using it this way protects them from the effects of frigid conditions.

CASE STUDY

Acute Injury

Uwe B. suffered a deep burn on the nail bed of his left thumb and complained of severe pain. It was a third-degree burn and about 8 mm in diameter. I advised him to put an adhesive bandage on the burn and told him which geometric figure to draw on the bandage. (See chapter 4 for how to determine which symbol to use.) The pain was alleviated at once. Uwe B. showed me his thumb after a week had gone by and reported a pain-free course of healing. The burn was completely healed, with no scar left behind.

THE SYMBOL
OF ELECTROSMOG
REDUCING THE POLLUTION
OF ELECTROSMOG

This symbol, which is reminiscent of an I Ching sign, consists of a special combination of lines and is mainly used for electrosmog and geological radiation pollution. To discharge this type of energy from the body, simply gaze upon this sign for a few minutes. The symbol can be placed on electrical devices like cell phones and computers to free them of interference from this kind of pollution.

3

Testing the Resonance Principle

Using a Single-Handed Dowsing Rod

The simplest tool for identifying resonance is a single-handed dowsing rod, also called a tensor. This magic wand of the modern age is easy to use and requires no previous knowledge or psychic talent. The most common rods now come in a variety of grip sizes and often include

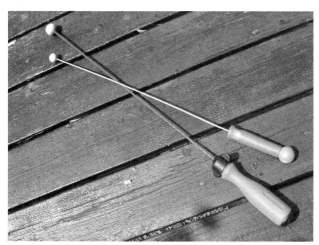

Single-handed dowsing rods, or tensors

a wooden ball at the tip, which many practitioners have found to be helpful. From our experience this one-handed rod is indeed a wonderfully simple and well-functioning tensor. However, many other newly developed models made from different materials (rock crystal, for example) and of differing dimensions are also available and perfectly suited to the task. Simple pendulums are also effective. Whenever possible students should try out different tools to see which ones work best for them.

INDIVIDUAL CALIBRATION

Before you can use a one-handed rod properly, you must calibrate it to your individual settings. If you are right-handed, take the rod in your right hand; if you're left-handed, pick it up with your left. Now imagine a wonderful scene in your mind's eye—for example, a gorgeous sunset or a peaceful beach—and with all of your emotion think or say something positive and vitalizing, such as "super, super, super—yes, yes, yes!" It is important to observe the first movement of the rod. Is it a horizontal motion or a vertical one? Next think of something negative or unpleasant and watch the rod move in the opposite plane.

All subsequent work in informational medicine is built upon this simple testing procedure—the ability to distinguish positive and nega-

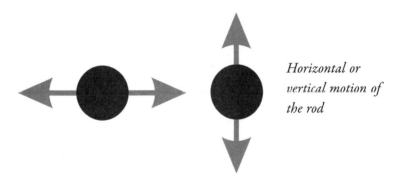

Horizontal or vertical motion of the rod

tive energies. It is best to learn this test procedure in a class, where you will receive many tips on the correct handling of the one-handed rod and have the opportunity for a good deal of practice. Such practice is necessary to build your confidence in the testing procedure and in your abilities.

To practice, place test objects in your non-dominant hand, or point to the object with your non-dominant index finger. Then observe the motion of the rod: it will indicate "wholesome" or "unwholesome," according to the horizontal or vertical schema you determined during your individual calibration. You can test the wholesomeness of foods, cosmetics, detergents, water, and so forth to gain practice.

The Classic Apple Exercise

For novices with the rod, the apple test is an ideal practice. Take a good fresh organic apple in your non-dominant hand and see which way your rod moves. Put the good apple down, then point to a rotten spot on another apple with your index finger: the motion of the rod should at once indicate an unwholesomeness.

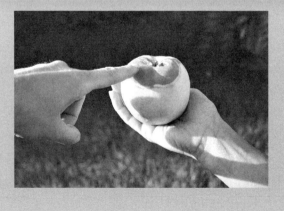

EVALUATING YOUR ABILITY TO TEST

Before each test you should do two things:

- open yourself mentally
- ascertain your own ability to test

Both steps are equally important for accurate testing. To accomplish the first step, practice gentle exercises, visualizations, breathing techniques, or simple meditations to open your heart and mind and connect you to the universe. Try to alleviate stress and connect the two hemispheres of your brain. Imagine yourself under a shower of gold that purifies you of everything that in any way negatively pollutes you.

When working with patients you will want to help them attune as well. It may be helpful to create a "healing image" for them, which might consist of watching themselves walk through an open door, for example, in order to symbolically begin the healing work. When the therapeutic work is concluded they walk their imaginary selves back through the door and close it behind them.

Once you have opened and attuned yourself, you can begin to evaluate your own testing ability with three short pre-tests.

1. Testing the Right and Left Hemispheres of the Brain

This test discerns the level of clarity of the right and left hemispheres of your brain, as well as the level of connection between them.

Hold your left hand (for left-handers, the right hand) a few centimeters (an inch or two) away from the right hemisphere of your brain. Hold the rod in a relaxed way in your other hand, and see which way it moves. Repeat this procedure with your hand a few centimeters away from the left hemisphere of your brain. The tip of the rod should have a positive indication in both instances.

If the rod does not give a positive reading, you do not have the ability to test at the moment. You should then draw one or two lines with your thumbnail from one side of your head to the other, going over the crown. If you test again the rod should have a positive movement. This procedure connects the two hemispheres of the brain and makes you able to test for about twenty minutes.

2. Testing the Back of the Head

Now test at the back of your head in the same way. This test evaluates your psychic state of mind in the moment.

If you are in a position to test, you will have a positive movement of the rod. If the movement of the rod is negative, draw two parallel lines with a fingernail along the midline of your head, from the crown to the nape of your neck. When you retest you should now have a positive movement and can perform further tests for about twenty minutes.

3. Testing the Top of the Head

This test looks for interference from electrosmog and geological radiation.

Hold your index finger or the palm of your hand over the highest point of your head. (This is the acupuncture point GV 20; see the figure on the following page.) You have testing ability when the rod provides a positive reading. If the rod provides a clearly negative reading, a geopathic disturbance is present—pollution due to geological radiation. On the other hand, a rotating reaction from the rod indicates electrosmog pollution. With a rotating or negative response from the rod, your ability to test accurately will be impaired. In either case change your location or look at the electrosmog symbol (see page 18) for a few minutes and do a retest. The movement of the rod should then be a positive one.

If you have obtained testing ability in this way, you can assume that your ability will remain for fifteen to thirty minutes.

GV 20

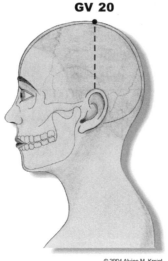

© 2004 Alvina M. Kreipl

The acupuncture point GV 20 is at the highest point on your head.

TESTING WITHOUT INTENTION

Expectations and preprogramming can influence the result of these subtle tests, so it is important to clear yourself of any specific intentions or desires before you begin your work. For instance, if you know that a patient has amalgam fillings, you should not expect that testing will show the fillings to be a negative influence: It could be that this patient is tolerating the amalgam well for the moment, or that other problems simply need to be addressed first. Perhaps the amalgam will show up in one of the coming sessions—or not.

Even in scientific research, it is understood that an underlying desire to obtain a certain result can influence the experimental process. The concept of a double-blind study—in which neither the doctor nor the patient knows which is the active agent and which is a placebo—was devised to avoid this influence. In order to be able to test without intentions we do not have to be blindfolded; we just need to remain relaxed and unbiased. Admittedly this is not so easy. We are so constantly inundated with information that our brains have installed many pigeonholes, in which we store preconceived notions, judgments, and prejudices. These preconceived ideas help us to process new information relatively quickly, but they also lead us to think first and then see.

In order to test without intention we need to reverse this programming and put ourselves in the condition of being present: first see, then think! We must be attentive and allow things to speak for themselves. Only in the here and now do we overcome schematic ways of thinking and render ourselves open to everything.

Important: Develop Confidence!

In working with the one-handed dowsing rod it is not only important to test without prejudice; you also have to develop confidence in your own testing results. If you are plagued by doubts about whether your test results are correct, you should keep practicing. In this work, as in all other disciplines, practice makes perfect!

Don't confuse perfection with absolute predictability, though. You may get different test results on different days with regard to the same query; for example, a particular food or medicine might test positive on some days and negative on others. In such cases you should write up your test results and ascertain any trend.

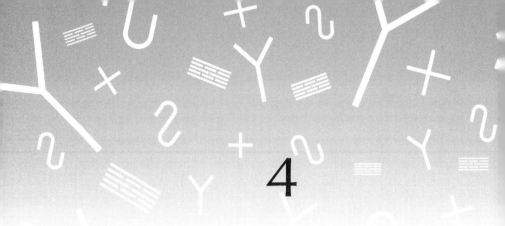

4

The Energy Circle

Testing and Balancing Energetic Influences

Having learned to use the one-handed dowsing rod, we are now able to test all influences around us for their wholesomeness or unwholesomeness in relation to our unique biosystem. Up to this point, however, we have learned only how to discern *whether* a food, a drug, a stone, or a thought is wholesome and harmonious for us or whether it is not.

The next level of practice with the rod will allow you to ascertain *how* wholesome a given food is for you, *how harmful* poisonous substances or heavy metals are for your organism, and *how vigorously* you should respond to a negative influence.

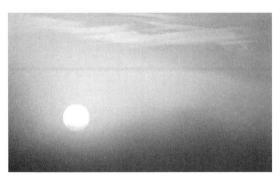

We are in constant exchange with our environment.

EXPANDING OUR TESTING POSSIBILITIES

Every vibration, regardless of whether it comes from the pollen of a flower or from a negative thought, has its characteristic wavelength and its very own informational content. This vibrational information can be measured according to the yes/no principle that we have already explored, and it can also be evaluated in terms of its gradations. We can look at these gradations through the energy circle.

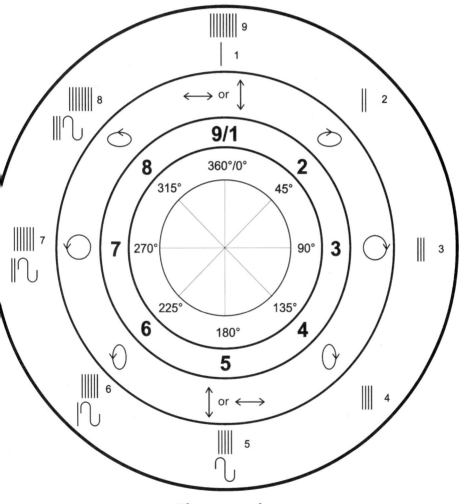

The energy circle

The energy circle indicates the degree of wholesomeness or the degree of severity of the pollution—without regard to whether the influence originated outside the body or within it. The lines, sine curves, and combination symbols associated with each section of the circle are then used to alter the vibrations that engage us so that they once more become wholesome for our biosystem. Whether we look at the symbols, paint them on our bodies, or attach them to some external object, they help to bring the "disturbing" vibration back into harmony with our own physical vibration. We will then be once more "on the same wavelength" with the world around us.

In this way the energy circle is simultaneously an instrument of diagnosis—in that every movement of the rod indicates something about the condition of the person in question—and an instrument of therapy, in that the symbol assigned to each code of the circle is an emblem for harmonizing the blockage.

CASE STUDY
Wound Healing

Petra S. came to me with a severe laceration. She had accidentally cut her hand between the lower and middle joint of her middle finger, removing a piece of skin 5 mm in size and 3 mm deep. The wound caused severe pain, and she felt a strong throbbing at the wound site. I put an adhesive bandage on the finger and painted the appropriate symbol—as tested out by the energy circle—on the bandage.

Almost immediately Petra S. reported that the throbbing pain had eased. I recommended that she redraw the symbol on the bandage each time she changed the dressing for the next seven to ten days. After ten days she showed me her finger and reported a practically pain-free course of healing. The piece of skin that had been removed was completely restored, and four weeks later the laceration was fully healed with no remaining scar.

THE EIGHT LEVELS OF WHOLESOMENESS

The energy circle is divided into eight sections that correspond to eight levels or gradations of wholesomeness. Each section is associated with a distinct movement of the dowsing rod and with a distinct sign or "bar code" for its remedy.

Grade 1: Undisturbed Wholesomeness

This grade, which demonstrates absolutely undisturbed harmonious and fluid balance, is indicated by the positive "yes" movement of your rod—which will be either a straight vertical or a straight horizontal motion, according to how you have defined "wholesomeness" during your initial calibration.

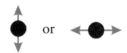

Note that our energy circle illustration shows a horizontal motion at grade 1 and a vertical movement as its opposite, grade 5. If your positive motion is vertical, simply change the grade 1 sign to a vertical image and the grade 5 sign to a horizontal one; all the other grades remain the same.

In the circle, grade 1 is shown at 0°/360°. The assigned symbol is a single line.

Grade 2: Very Limited Pollution

The tensor will indicate this grade with a clockwise elliptical motion, describing a sideways oval. In the diagram of the circle, grade 2 is shown at 45°. The assigned symbol is two parallel lines.

Grade 3: Minor Degree of Pollution

The tensor indicates this grade with a clockwise circular motion. In the energy circle, grade 3 is shown at 90°. The assigned symbol is three parallel lines.

Grade 4: Medium Pollution

The tensor indicates this grade by describing an upstanding oval turning clockwise. In the energy circle, grade 4 is shown at 135°. The assigned symbol is four parallel lines.

Grade 5: Unwholesome

This is your "no" movement, unwholesome as you have determined it. So if your tensor showed a horizontal movement at grade 1, grade 5 will be indicated by a vertical movement. If you use a vertical movement at grade 1, on the other hand, then grade 5 will be horizontal for you. In the circle, grade 5 is shown at 180°—exactly opposite the perfectly balanced grade 1. The assigned symbol can be either five parallel lines or the sine curve—the sign of reversal.

Grade 6: Severe Pollution

The tensor indicates this grade by drawing an upright oval turning counterclockwise. In the energy circle, grade 6 is shown at 225°. The assigned symbol is six parallel lines or one line plus a sine curve.

Grade 7: Very Severe Pollution

The tensor indicates this grade with a counterclockwise circle. In the energy circle diagram, grade 7 is shown at 270°. The assigned symbol is either seven parallel lines or two parallel lines plus a sine curve.

Grade 8: Extremely Severe Pollution

The tensor indicates this grade with a sideways oval turning counterclockwise. In the energy circle, grade 8 is shown at 315°. The assigned symbol is eight parallel lines or three parallel lines plus the sine curve.*

||||||| *Grade 9*

The tensor indicates the same movement and vibrates in the same direction as it does for grade 1, but its motions are somewhat stronger. At this grade, the circle is closed. Its end is simultaneously the beginning of a new cycle; death is also rebirth. From this philosophical perspective, it is logical that the rod's motion would be the same at grade 9 as at grade 1; 360° = 0°. The stronger movement that denotes grade 9, however, indicates that we are now at the next higher level of vibration.

In the energy circle grade 9 is at 360°. The assigned symbol is nine parallel lines. In practice, the nine lines usually have special functions: they are not used like the other symbols to reverse unwholesomeness. A full discussion of their use, however, is advanced work that is beyond the scope of this book.

> *This must ye ken!*
> *From one take ten;*
> *Skip two and then*
> *Even up three.*
> *And rich you'll be.*
> *Leave out the four.*
> *From five and six,*
> *Thus says the witch,*

---

*The energy circle is a theoretical working model. In practice a very severe pollution, such as the one expressed at grade 8, almost never occurs. Even if you were to ascertain pollution of this kind, the symbol for grade 7 would be sufficient to restore the energetic balance. To be certain you would ask, "Is two lines + sine curve sufficient for balance?" If a "yes" comes, accept it, because three lines + sine curve (or eight lines) might possibly overtax the organism.

> *Make seven and eight,*
> *And all is straight.*
> *And nine is one,*
> *And ten is none.*
> *This, the witch's one-time-one!*
> —*Goethe*, Faust *Part I*
>
> Johann Wolfgang von Goethe, the author of this poem, already knew, or felt, that I and 9 have the same vibration . . .

In general all indications of the rod turning in a clockwise direction— that is, up to grade 4—indicate that the organism (body, soul, and spirit) is still in a position to help itself. Because everything vibrates, much of the blockage can be overcome by the ordinary course of events.

From grade 5 onward, however, our biosystems will generally be unable to emerge from the blockage on their own, and will require a healing impulse. All counterclockwise movements of the rod indicate a condition in need of treatment, which can be effected with the associated symbols. These "bar codes" are extremely varied in their usage and can reverse a wide range of unwholesome information, including allergies, illnesses, bleeding, negative dogmas, and so on. More information on working with specific conditions will be found in the following chapters.

When you have mastered the use of the energy circle with the one-handed dowsing rod, you will be able to discover the correct healing symbol without much trouble. To hone your skills and develop greater confidence, we recommend that you take a dowsing or basic New Homeopathy class in which the model of the energy circle is demonstrated and practiced.

Practice Makes Perfect

With the help of the energy circle, practice the oval and circular movements of the rod. Impress upon yourself the movement that corresponds to each level of pollution and the sign of harmonization assigned to it. For example, when you get a circling movement to the left, you should be able to remember that a leftward circle indicates grade 7. You know that pollution at the level of grade 7 is rather severe. The sign that can provide a healing impulse would here be ‖∩U.

It is important that you pay attention to the way the question is posed! Make sure to be specific, and ask questions like "How unwholesome is this apple for me?" or "How severe is the pollution?" and so forth. If you simply ask "Is this apple good for me?" the answer you receive will not give you a clear remedy.

CASE STUDY

Protection from Mosquitos

I spent my summer vacation on Corfu, where at night there were swarms of mosquitos. When I arrived in my hotel room I counted four or five mosquitos and I immediately affixed the mosquito net I'd obtained especially for this vacation over the bed. Since the buzzing of mosquitos tends to keep me awake, I also decided to use my energy-painting practices to clear the room.

To begin, I tested the wholesomeness of the room with the energy circle. Then I drew the sign that had been indicated by the test on a piece of paper. I also wrote on this paper the name of the building, the room number, and the word "mosquito." I placed this piece of paper in the middle of the room.

After a few minutes I ventilated the room and most of the mosquitos flew outside; others flew right toward me and I could kill them. My room was then free of mosquitos. After about six days I suddenly again had five mosquitos in my room. I tested my piece of paper again, but this time the sign that I'd used previously tested too high. I used a somewhat weaker symbol and slept in a mosquito-free room for the rest of my vacation.

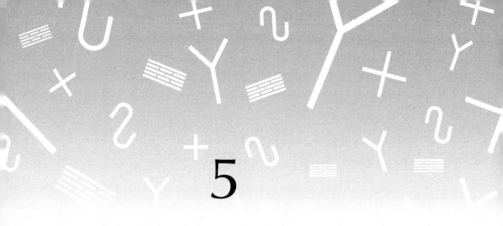

5

The Energy Balance

Regulating Energy in the Body with
Chinese Medicine

While there are many ways and many systems of describing energy in the body, New Homeopathy and its practices often make use of the energy terminology of Chinese medicine. The clear maps and sophisticated energetic relationships described by Chinese medicine help to identify areas and specific points of imbalance in the body.

While acupuncture needling has become widely known in Western culture as a therapeutic method for harmonizing or restoring the flow of energy, the energy painting methods described in this book allow people who do not like needles to receive effective therapy and restore harmonious flow in their meridians. Experience shows that symbols and bar codes drawn on acupuncture points possess a healing power equal to that of the acupuncture needles.

Below is a brief introduction to some of the foundational concepts of Chinese medicine, and the ways that the meridian system can be adapted to painting the energy body. The theory of the five phases of transformation is especially helpful in the way it shows us how everything is interconnected with everything else, and how important it is to allow each element to have its space so that no single one can be overly powerful.

THE POLARITY PRINCIPLE
YIN AND YANG

We have seen that everything around us is in a state of vibration and that movement occurs in the interplay between the two poles—positive and negative. This principle of life is an ancient law recognized in many cultures. In Chinese philosophy this polarity is described by the principle of yin and yang. Disease, in this model, arises from conditions of "fullness" and "emptiness" in the energetic streams that comprise the organs and meridians. Erich Körbler, too, saw disease as a disturbed balance in the energy system, the blockage of which is defined by insufficient energy or information.

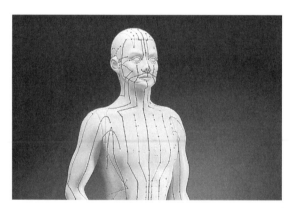

Disease is defined by energy blockages or disturbances in the meridian system.

Yin and yang are two polarities, a pairing that is more about complements than it is about opposites. For without the night there would be no day, as it is the night that releases the coming day. We only feel joy because we also know sadness. Yang is the masculine principle, yin the feminine one—these are complementary values, free of judgment. The one can be nothing without the other, nor is one "right" or the other "wrong." As the male organism also produces female hormones, we can see that within the male principle a kernel of the feminine exists, and vice versa. In spite of the appearance of duality everything is ONE.

The monad: symbol of yin and yang. The opposing poles both contain their opposites.

EXAMPLES OF YIN AND YANG

Yin	Yang
Feminine	Masculine
Material	Energy
Round	Angular
Night	Day
Moon	Sun
Earth	Sky
Winter	Summer
Receiving Principle	Giving Principle
Passive	Active
Wet	Dry
Inner	Outer
Rest	Movement
Soft	Forceful
Inhalation	Exhalation
Storage Organs	Hollow Organs
Parasympathetic System	Sympathetic System
Degenerative Diseases	Acute Diseases

THE FIVE PHASES OF TRANSFORMATION

In addition to the yin/yang polarity of all being, the theory of the five phases of transformation—also known as the doctrine of the five elements—is basic to the philosophy of the Chinese system of healing. According to this theory all phenomena of humanity and the environment are ordered according to five basic stages of evolution: wood, fire, earth, metal, and water. These five phases of transformation underlie a constant dynamic: They mutually bring each other forth, control one another, and are mutually interdependent. If one element is too heavily emphasized, another will be automatically weakened. A healthy organism is distinguished by the fact that the five elements nourish and control each other mutually, and thus the organism (by which is meant the unity of body, soul, and spirit) exists in a harmonious balance.

The Sheng Cycle: Circulation of Nourishment

None of the five elements can exist without the others: each element creates and "nourishes" the next one. In Chinese philosophy this is the concept of the nourishment of the child by its mother.

- Wood nourishes fire, because fire needs wood to burn.
- Fire nourishes earth, because earth arises from ashes.
- Earth nourishes metal, because metal comes from the earth.
- Metal nourishes water, because water condenses on metal.
- Water nourishes wood, because wood cannot grow without water.

After one "go-around" the circulation of life is not concluded in any final way, it simply begins again. Just as after death life begins again, the last element inevitably brings forth the first one again. All of being is a constant circulation without beginning or end, and every child is at the same time the mother of the next element.

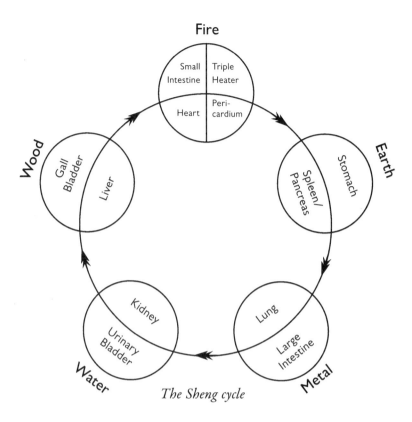

The Sheng cycle

Example of the Sheng Cycle

The upward-striving power of childhood is ascribed to the young, green tree (wood element). In this phase we want to broaden our horizons. We learn to channel our forceful desire toward success within certain limits. If support is lacking here, perhaps because the mother (water) was weak, frustration arises and vitality suffers: aggression is often the result. This mental condition is then drawn into the fire element—into an adult condition—where it can get into overly "heated" situations such as a desire for conflict or high blood pressure (heart).

The Ko Cycle: Control

The elements wood, fire, earth, metal, and water not only nourish one another, they can also mutually control each other. The goal is to keep one element from becoming too powerful and disturbing the system's balance. In Chinese medicine the Ko cycle corresponds to the control of a child by its grandmother, for in Chinese society the grandmother has a much stronger level of participation in the upbringing of a child than in our culture.

The control system can be understood as follows:

- Wood controls earth, just as a wooden plow splits the earth.
- Earth controls water, for a dike holds a river back.
- Water controls fire, for water extinguishes fire.
- Fire controls metal, for fire causes metal to melt.
- Metal controls wood, for a hatchet splits wood.

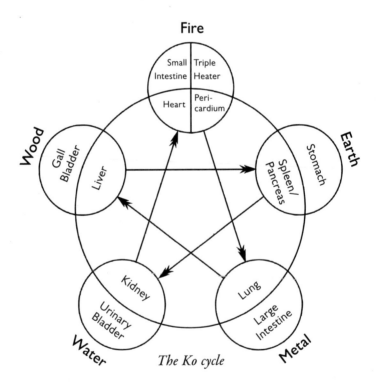

The Ko cycle

The Overpowering Cycle

If the "grandson" becomes overly powerful within the control cycle, we say that it "rebels" against the grandmother. The element that is actually supposed to be controlled acquires the upper hand. This process is called the overpowering cycle: Earth overpowers wood, so that the wooden plow breaks. Wood overpowers metal, so that the hatchet breaks. Metal overpowers fire, so that the fire is smothered by metal. Fire overpowers water, so that the extinguishing water is insufficient. Water overpowers earth, so that the dike breaks.

The doctrine of five elements describes still other cycles, but going deeper into them would lead us too far astray here. The essence of this system is the principle that everything is connected to everything else: all things in life depend on each other, and an excess or deficiency of one aspect results in an imbalance that unavoidably affects the collective interaction in a negative way. This can happen on a spiritual, psychological, or physical level. The consistent aim of all healing efforts is the rebalancing of the system, which we effect in New Homeopathy with the inscription of symbols on acupuncture points.

The description of the five phases of transformation should provide you with an impression of how important it is to maintain—or rebuild—balance on all levels. But do not worry about memorizing all of this information; the practical work of the inscription of the bar codes can be done without knowing the five elements by heart.

ORGAN/MERIDIAN CORRESPONDENCES

Each of the five elements is associated with a pair of meridians, which in turn consists of a yin and a yang organ.* These "organs" are understood more broadly than Western culture's definition of a limited cluster

---

*Unlike the other elements, the fire element actually consists of two organ pairs—the Heart and Small Intestine and the Pericardium and Triple Heater.

of anatomical cells: instead, TCM organs are understood as energetic entities with definite functions that mutually influence one another. Together, the twelve organs and their meridians govern and direct the body's many processes. When the organs are acting in harmony with each other, the body, mind, and spirit are healthy and filled with vitality. When one or more organs are out of balance, symptoms and diseases will arise.

Element	Wood	Fire	Earth	Metal	Water
Organ/ meridian	Liver (yin), Gall Bladder (yang)	Heart (yin), Small Intestine (yang), Pericardium (yin), Triple Heater (yang)	Spleen/ Pancreas (yin), Stomach (yang)	Lungs (yin), Large Intestine (yang)	Kidney (Yin), Urinary Bladder (yang)
Age	Childhood	Adolescence	Adulthood	Middle Age	Old Age
Season	Spring	Summer	Late Summer	Fall	Winter
Color	Green	Red	Yellow/ brown	White	Blue/ black
Sense	Sight	Speech	Taste	Smell	Hearing
Emotion	Anger	Joy	Sympathy	Sorrow/ grief	Fear
Tissue	Muscles, sinews, joints	Blood vessels	Connective tissue	Skin	Bones
Taste	Sour	Bitter	Sweet	Pungent	Salty

FUNCTIONS OF THE ORGANS AND MERIDIANS

Below is a brief description of each of the twelve organs and their main functions. The meridian associated with each organ traverses a specific part of the body and helps to connect it to the other organs and meridians. Each of the meridians has one or more points that are particularly well-suited for treatment with the healing symbols; a brief description and a guide to locating these particular points can be found at the end of each section.

The Liver Meridian (Yin Wood)

The Liver meridian is perceived as a "general," who supervises events and issues sensible commands. Associated with the eyes and vision, the Liver also governs foresight and the ability to plan. It controls the smooth flow of energy—both physical and emotional—and strengthens the defense function. The Liver also influences the composition of the blood.

- *Negative emotions of the Liver:* anger, small-mindedness, not being able to see the big picture.
- *Psychological purpose of the Liver:* ability to let emotions come and go, not becoming attached to them.

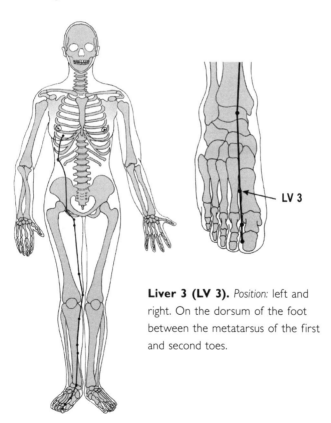

Liver 3 (LV 3). *Position:* left and right. On the dorsum of the foot between the metatarsus of the first and second toes.

The Gall Bladder Meridian (Yang Wood)

According to the plans of the Liver, the Gall Bladder converts decisions sensibly into fact. The Gall Bladder stands for courage and bravery and for a healthy sense of justice. This includes the ability to say things that other people do not like and the ability to take action when others are hesitating.

- *Negative emotions of the Gall Bladder:* indecision, lacking a sense of justice, indifference, lack of dependability, lack of punctuality.

- *Psychological purpose of the Gall Bladder:* a healthy power of discernment, a good feel for the correctness of things, enterprise.

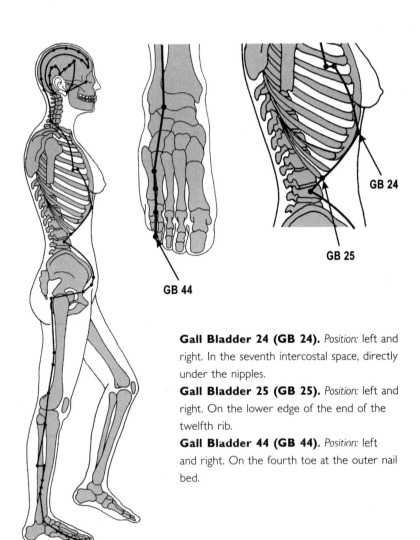

GB 24

GB 25

GB 44

Gall Bladder 24 (GB 24). *Position:* left and right. In the seventh intercostal space, directly under the nipples.

Gall Bladder 25 (GB 25). *Position:* left and right. On the lower edge of the end of the twelfth rib.

Gall Bladder 44 (GB 44). *Position:* left and right. On the fourth toe at the outer nail bed.

The Heart Meridian (Yin Fire)

The Heart is a person's spiritual center. It is the ruler of the other organs, and is sometimes called the "prince of fire." The heart and Heart meridian guide the circulation of the blood, the brain, the five senses, the emotions, and thought.

- *Negative emotions of the Heart:* nervousness, restlessness, quick fatigue, nervous exhaustion, insomnia, emotional imbalance, stress.

- *Psychological purpose of the Heart:* balance of the emotions, clear thought that is expressed with a clear manner of speech, awareness in leading your life, a healthy perception of the harmony between heaven and earth.

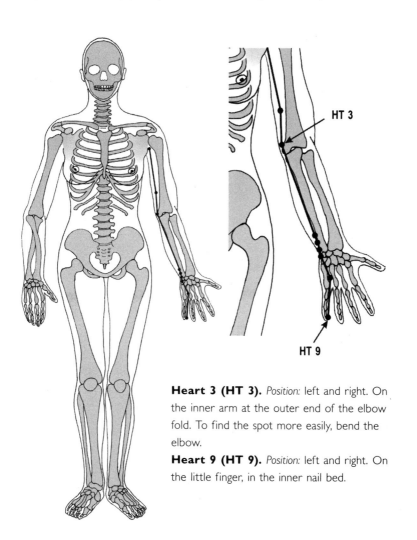

Heart 3 (HT 3). *Position:* left and right. On the inner arm at the outer end of the elbow fold. To find the spot more easily, bend the elbow.

Heart 9 (HT 9). *Position:* left and right. On the little finger, in the inner nail bed.

The Small Intestine Meridian (Yang Fire)

The Small Intestine guides the distribution of nutrients to the whole organism. Alongside this material purpose, the Small Intestine also has the function of "digesting" thoughts and impulses from the environment, instead of simply accepting knowledge or strange convictions in an unprocessed state.

- *Negative emotions of the Small Intestine:* hypersensitivity, anxiety, depression, unclear thought.

- *Psychological purpose of the Small Intestine:* reception of the thoughts of others and one's own experiences and their healthy digestion, rejection and sorting out of psychologically indigestible things, formation of one's own view of the world.

Small Intestine 3 (SI 3). *Position:* left and right. With the hand in a loose fist, the point on the outside edge of the palm, at the end of the most prominent palm line.

Small Intestine 8 (SI 8). *Position:* left and right. On the inner arm, at the outermost point of the elbow crease, in the depression between the ulna and the humerus.

Small Intestine 19 (SI 19). *Position:* right side only. In front of the ear, in the depression between the tragus and the jawbone when the mouth is slightly open.

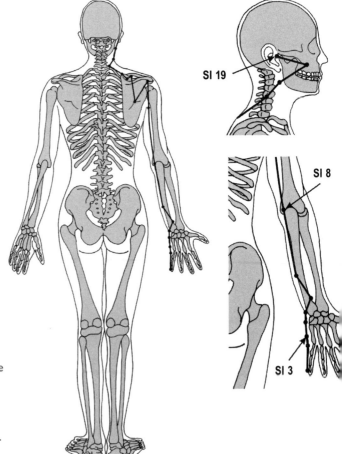

SI 19

SI 8

SI 3

The Pericardium Meridian (Yin Fire)

The Pericardium is the protector of the heart and is often called the Heart Protector. Its functions are very similar to those of the heart: guiding the coronary blood vessels along with the rest of the circulatory system. The Pericardium also influences the digestion and delivers energy for the sexual organs.

- *Negative emotions of the Pericardium:* hypersensitivity, frequent anxiety, disturbance of concentration, spiritual aloofness, insomnia, feelings of anxiety, restriction in the chest cavity.

- *Psychological purpose of the Pericardium:* to be able to open one's self with kindness toward others and toward one's partner, to develop depth and warmth in love and sexuality.

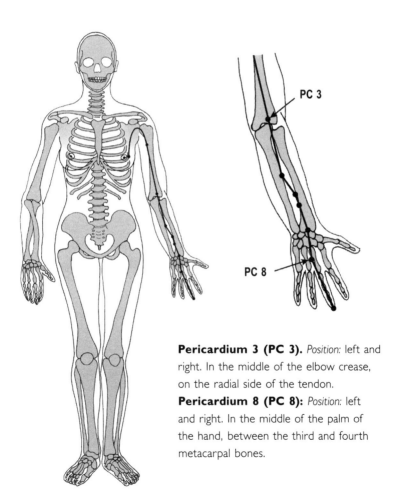

Pericardium 3 (PC 3). *Position:* left and right. In the middle of the elbow crease, on the radial side of the tendon.
Pericardium 8 (PC 8): *Position:* left and right. In the middle of the palm of the hand, between the third and fourth metacarpal bones.

The Triple Heater (Yang Fire)

Traditional Chinese medicine includes the concept of three combustion chambers in the body, which are known collectively as the Triple Heater. The upper heater sits in the chest cavity and influences breath, the middle heater is situated approximately in the region of the stomach and influences digestion, and the lower heater is in the lower abdomen and pelvis and influences sexuality and the excretory functions. The Triple Heater coordinates and regulates these three functions and also protects against influences from the outside. It is sometimes known as the "foreign minister."

- *Negative emotions of the Triple Heater:* hypersensitivity to cold, wind, and dampness; exaggerated cautiousness; nervous excitement; sleep disorders; obsessions; limited ability to cope with emotional changes (e.g., travel).

- *Psychological purpose of the Triple Heater:* development of a healthy protective mechanism against influences of all kinds—in the physical, psychological, and social arenas—inner balance, knowledge as to when it is time to lead and when it is time to step back.

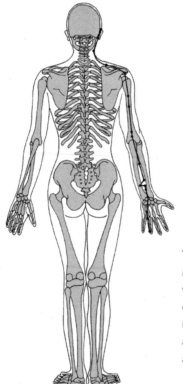

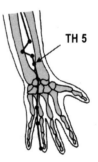

TH 5

Triple Heater 5 (TH 5).
Position: left and right. Where the wristwatch normally sits: in the depression between the ulna and radius on the outside of the lower arm, about two finger-breadths above the fold of the wrist.

The Spleen/Pancreas (Yin Earth)

The Spleen/Pancreas is the main organ of digestion in Chinese medicine, transforming the foods we eat into energy, and transporting that energy to the other organs that require it. It also plays an important role in immunity through the lymphatic system and helps to build blood. It is connected with digestion, energy, and menstruation.

- *Negative emotions of the Spleen/Pancreas:* general weakness, too much worry, brooding, forgetfulness, unrest in the legs, insufficient concentration, craving for sweets, eating disorders/psychological conflicts that are not about the satisfaction of hunger but about feeling unable to cope with the senselessness of life in a materially "over-satiated" world.

- *Psychological purpose of the Spleen/Pancreas:* ability to care about someone, to take over care and responsibility, the position of the "mediator" between the creative universe and terrestrial fertility, realization of the maternal, nurturing principle, care for harmonious interpersonal relationships.

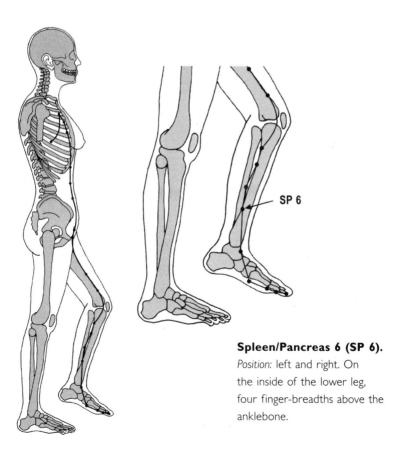

SP 6

Spleen/Pancreas 6 (SP 6).
Position: left and right. On the inside of the lower leg, four finger-breadths above the anklebone.

The Stomach (Yang Earth)

The main function of the Stomach consists of the intake of nourishment and its preparation for the transmission into the small intestine. In a broad sense the Stomach absorbs not only material nourishment but also our experiences and the things we learn. It decides whether we can "digest" difficult situations or whether we must react, for example, by developing a stomach ulcer.

- *Negative emotions of the Stomach:* refusal to take in the world, rebellion, feelings of overwhelm, a tendency to retreat from daily tasks.

- *Psychological purpose of the Stomach:* formation of a fruitful relationship with mother and father, development of a natural "taste" (in clothing, furniture, loving preparation of food, etc.), permission and active ability to take what one needs or would like to have.

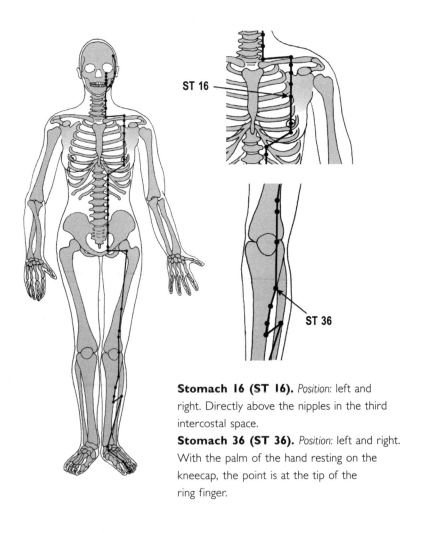

Stomach 16 (ST 16). *Position:* left and right. Directly above the nipples in the third intercostal space.
Stomach 36 (ST 36). *Position:* left and right. With the palm of the hand resting on the kneecap, the point is at the tip of the ring finger.

The Lungs (Yin Metal)

The Lungs absorb fundamental energy—the basic life force called chi, ki, or prana—from the atmosphere. The Lungs inhale this pure energy and exhale its waste products. They also govern our resistance to diseases from the outside. The central theme of the Lungs is the natural back-and-forth of life, exemplified in the process of breathing, in which we unload waste and take in new energy in a constant exchange.

- *Negative emotions of the Lungs:* inadequate vitality, loss of strength, weak borders between one's self and the environment, vulnerability and hyper-sensitivity, inability to accept consolation; concealment, repression of sorrow.

- *Psychological purpose of the Lungs:* to find structure in life, develop stability, balance between near and far, ability to distance one's self internally, and to be able to reflect on and rework events, and to learn to accept consolation.

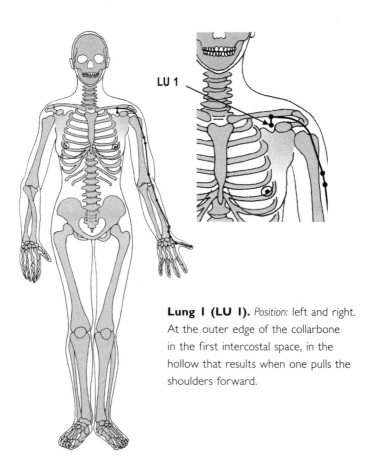

LU 1

Lung 1 (LU 1). *Position:* left and right. At the outer edge of the collarbone in the first intercostal space, in the hollow that results when one pulls the shoulders forward.

The Large Intestine (Yang Metal)

The Large Intestine takes in the remnants of nourishment from the Small Intestine and sorts out the waste materials. It divides the impure from the pure and allows to pass what is of no use to us. It can get out of balance through incorrect nourishment, weakness, or agitation. The function of the Large Intestine is closely tied to the idea of "letting go," which is absent when we are constipated, for example.

- *Negative emotions of the Large Intestine:* overweening desire to control, holding to old patterns, fear, delegation of responsibilities, insufficient trust in the flow of life.

- *Psychological purpose of the Large Intestine:* trusting in the natural flow of life, learning to let go, entrusting one's self to the constant exchange between intake and outflow, constantly dealing with and reflecting the process of life.

Large Intestine 1 (LI 1). *Position:* left and right. In the nail bed of the index finger, on the side nearest the thumb.

Large Intestine 11 (LI 11). *Position:* left and right. When the elbow is bent, the point is on the outside of the arm, at the end of the elbow crease.

Large Intestine 19 (LI 19). In New Homeopathy, this point is known as the "toxin point," and is considered to reflect the presence of heavy metals or other toxins in the body. *Position:* right side only. Beneath/ beside the nostril.

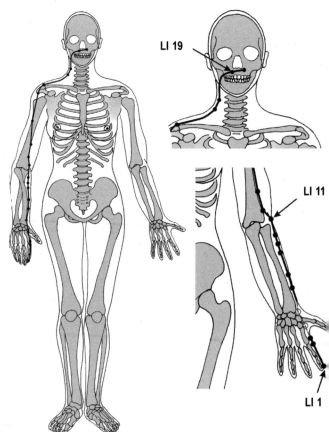

The Kidneys (Yin Water)

According to Chinese medicine, the Kidneys "store" the experiential energy of our ancestors and deliver that energy to all the other organs of the body. They are therefore largely responsible for our liveliness and the degree of our vitality. Just as water is necessary for all processes of life inside and outside the cells, the vital energy of the Kidneys is important for all the other processes of life. The Kidneys also influence sexual energy; therefore, an excessive or deficient level of sexual desire is connected to this organ.

- *Negative emotions of the Kidney:* exaggerated fears that have no relation to actual threats; panic, depression, rigidity, and immobility in thought and emotion; pessimistic attitude toward life; insufficient ability to decide things.

- *Psychological purpose of the Kidney:* getting into the flow of life, letting one's self be carried by the waves of the ocean, being tender, being able to abandon one's self and learn to trust the power of water.

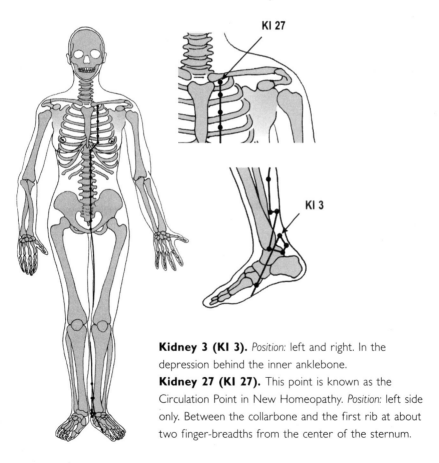

Kidney 3 (KI 3). *Position:* left and right. In the depression behind the inner anklebone.

Kidney 27 (KI 27). This point is known as the Circulation Point in New Homeopathy. *Position:* left side only. Between the collarbone and the first rib at about two finger-breadths from the center of the sternum.

The Urinary Bladder (Yang Water)

The Urinary Bladder guides the storage and elimination of urine that comes from the Kidneys; it is virtually the "governor" of the basic life energy that comes from the Kidneys. It takes care of correctly dividing the body's water, and making sure that it can neither oversaturate nor dry out different parts of the body. This meridian is therefore decisively responsible for the balance in our bodily fluids.

- *Negative emotions of the Urinary Bladder:* hypersensitivity and jumpiness to the point of fearfulness. Those afflicted tend toward nervousness, get aggravated easily over trifles, and have disturbing dreams.

- *Psychological purpose of the Urinary Bladder:* to be able to relax spiritually and physically, allowing inner quietude and spiritual rest.

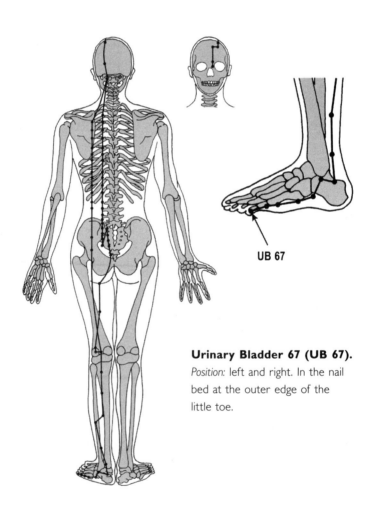

UB 67

Urinary Bladder 67 (UB 67).
Position: left and right. In the nail bed at the outer edge of the little toe.

THE ENERGY BALANCE PROCESS
PREPARATION AND PRACTICE

The bar code symbols can be placed on the meridian points described above to rebalance energy in the meridians or to release specific restrictions. Specific points on the body are tested with the tensor (see the table on page 60), and every point that indicates blockage is immediately balanced with a symbol on that point. This process is called the "energy balance." You can conduct an energy balance for yourself as well as for another person.

This system serves as a diagnostic tool, providing information about a person's balance or lack of energy, and it is also an immediate treatment for helping to remove blockages and improve imbalances. The testing procedure can help you to discover negative influences, both from the external environment—like electrosmog or geological radiation pollution—and from the internal environment, such as allergies from blood poisoning (mycosis) or pollution caused by dental amalgam.

Preliminary Tests

Before you can conduct an effective energy balance session, you first need to do some preliminary tests. In the following description we assume that the energy balance is being conducted for another person.

1. Examine the Ability to Test

Just as you tested yourself in chapter 3 for your ability to use the energy circle, you will test yourself and the person you are working with to be sure you can both test clearly. First test yourself on the following areas: left and right hemispheres of the brain, psychic situation of the moment (the back of the head), geopathic disturbance and electrosmog (crown of the head/GV 20). If need be, do the rebalancing lines to connect the two hemispheres of the brain as described in chapter 3, then test again to be sure that everything is in order.

After you have tested and cleared yourself, do the same for the person you are working with.

2. Spinal Column Reflexes on the Head

Just as certain zones of the feet or hands can be mapped to reflect the condition of the body's inner organs and systems, Erich Körbler determined that the top of the skull can reflect the energy of the spinal column and the organs connected to it. Proceeding from the highest point on the head (GV 20) along the top of the skull to the front hairline, we can test the energy situation of the spine and the organs connected to it.

With your non-dominant index finger, trace slowly along the midline of the head from GV 20 to the forehead, and observe the results shown by the tensor. If the tensor displays a negative reading during this process, make note of it. After you have performed the energy balance procedures, this disturbance should be gone.

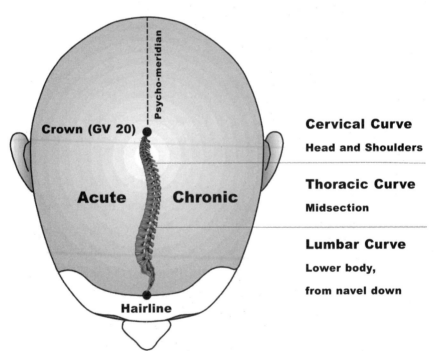

Reflection of the spinal column on the top of the skull

3. Testing the Spine

The third preliminary test concerns the spinal column itself. Gently run your non-dominant index finger down the spine, starting at the first vertebra and continuing all the way down to the sacrum. Note any places where the tensor shows a negative or imbalanced reading, and be sure to recheck them after the energy balance.

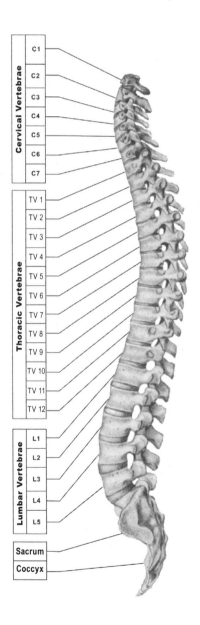

The spinal column

Equalizing the Meridians: Performing the
Energy Balance Procedure

In the chart on pages 60–61, you will see the most important acupuncture points and some additional test points for the performance of the energy balance. Most of the points are situated on the hands and feet. One test point is sufficient for each meridian, as it reflects and harmonizes the energy of the whole course of the meridian.

The tensor reading on these points will determine whether energetic blockages are present, weakening the body's energy system. In order to re-establish balance, the correct symbol should immediately be painted on the tested part of the body with a washable felt-tip or ballpoint pen (do not use a permanent marker). This simple remedy balances energetic deficits and releases blockages on the spot—in the meridian being worked on, and often also in adjacent meridians.

After the meridian points you will also test a few special points: the inflammation point, hormone/thyroid point, circulation point, blood fungus/mycosis point, heavy metals point, and allergies point. In the beginning you may think: "How am I supposed to remember this?" But do not fear: once you have performed the energy balance three to four times, you will know these points by heart. As with the other techniques discussed in this book, you will learn these practices most effectively if you can take a class in which the participants perform and practice the energy balance on each other.

1. Place your left index finger on the first point in the chart on page 60 and observe the movement of the tensor.
2. If the tensor shows a grade 5 or higher, draw the balancing bar code (as shown on the energy circle in chapter 4) on the location described in the last column of the table.
3. Retest after you have drawn the symbol, to see if the meridian has been balanced to grade 1. When it is balanced, go on to

the next test point—in this case the same point on the other hand—and proceed as before until all points have been tested and balanced.

4. Work thoroughly on both sides of the body, that is, Large Intestine 1 on the left and right index finger, Heart 9 on the left and right small finger, etc. Note that the additional test points described at the end of the chart are found on one side of the body only.

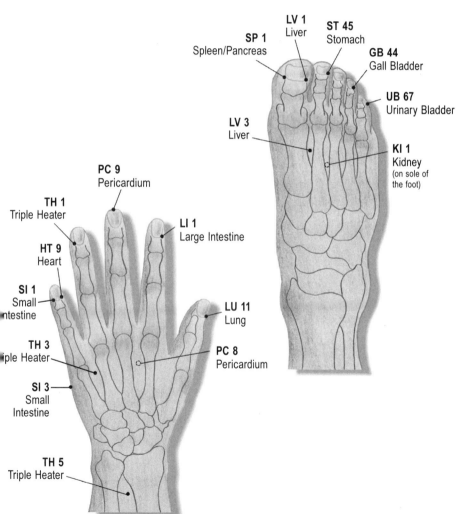

Test points on the hands and feet

THE POINTS OF THE TESTING SEQUENCE

Classical Acupuncture Points	Testing Location	Symbol Location
Large Intestine 1	Index finger, inner nail bed	LI 1 or LI 11 (Outside of the elbow fold)
Heart 9	Little finger, inner nail bed	HT 9 or HT 3 (Inside of the elbow fold)
Small Intestine 3	Outside hand—fold	SI 3 (Same position as test site)
Pericardium 8	Middle of the palm	PC 8 or PC 3 (Middle of the elbow fold)
Triple Heater 5	Middle of the outer wrist, where a wristwatch sits	TH 5 (Same position as the test site)
Lung 1	Angle of the collarbone and shoulder joint	LU 1 (Same position as the test site)
Liver 3	Top of the foot next to the base joint of the big toe	LV 3 (Same position as the test site)
Kidney 3	Depression behind the inner anklebone	KI 3 (Same position as the test site)
Spleen/Pancreas 6	4 finger-breadths above the inner ankle	SP 6 (Same position as the test site)
Stomach 36	Place the palm of the hand on the knee and guide the ring finger about 2 cm toward the outside beside the shinbone	ST 36 (Same position as the test site)
Gall Bladder 44	fourth toe (counted from the big toe, toenail on the outside, toward the little toe	GB 44 (Same position as the test site)
Urinary Bladder 67	Little toe, outer nail bed	UB 67 (Same position as the test site)

ADDITIONAL TEST POINTS

Point	Testing Location	Symbol Location
Inflammation	Inside the wrist	Beyond grade 5, always 4 lines across the entire wrist
Hormone/ Thyroid	Middle of the throat point just below the depression	(Same position as the test site)
Circulation	Left side only: angle of the sternum and collarbone	KI 27 left (Same position as the test site)
Blood Fungi	Go from the middle of the left collarbone straight in the direction of the sternum. The position is to the left in the third inter-rib space.	(Same position as the test site)
Heavy Metals/ Toxins LI 19	Below the right nostril	LI 19 right (Same position as the test site)
Allergies SI 19	Directly in front of the right ear	SI 19 right (Same position as the test site)

Abbreviations:

LI = Large Intestine meridian

HT = Heart meridian

SI = Small Intestine meridian

PC = Pericardium meridian

TH = Triple Heater meridian

LU = Lung meridian

LV = Liver meridian

KI = Kidney meridian

SP = Spleen/Pancreas meridian

ST= Stomach meridian

GB = Gall Bladder meridian

UB = Urinary Bladder meridian

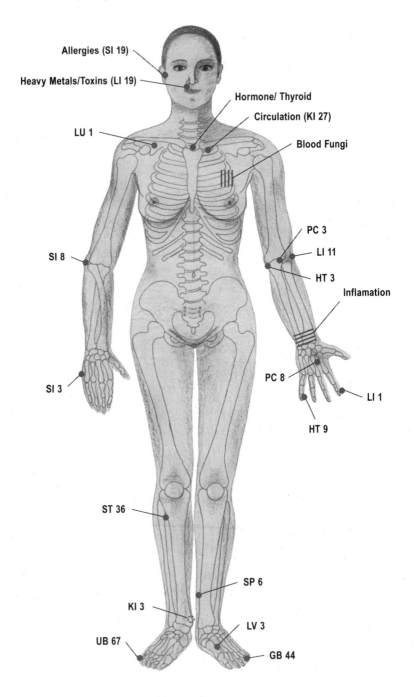

Allergies (SI 19)

Heavy Metals/Toxins (LI 19)

Hormone/ Thyroid

Circulation (KI 27)

LU 1

Blood Fungi

PC 3

LI 11

HT 3

SI 8

Inflamation

SI 3

PC 8

LI 1

HT 9

ST 36

SP 6

KI 3

LV 3

UB 67

GB 44

Additional test points

Determining the Length of Treatment

When you have completed the energy balance, you must determine how long each symbol should remain drawn on the body.

Place yourself next to the right shoulder* of the patient and put your left hand over the right hemisphere of the brain. Inquire how long the sign should remain on the body (hours, days). After this time the sign should be washed off so that the energy system does not react negatively (e.g., with unease or pain) when the energy frequency of the balancing sign no longer fits.

Special Considerations of the Additional Test Points

The additional test points work somewhat differently than the main meridian points, and should be treated as follows.

Inflammation Point

The four lines that are painted on the inflammation point connect the whole meridian system and increase immune defenses. You can use this symbol regardless of your energy status. If you have a cold or any inflammation, use the sign on this point to strengthen the immune system.

Hormone/Thyroid Point

The thyroid point concerns the whole hormonal system. In practice it has been shown that a sign usually needs to remain here for only a few minutes or a few hours; leaving it on too long can cause unease or other negative reactions in the patient. Therefore, test especially carefully for the duration of this treatment symbol.

Circulation Point (Kidney 27)

Test and balance the left side only (at the joint of the sternum and collarbone).

---

*Left-handed people should stand next to the patient's left shoulder and put their right hand over the left hemisphere of the brain.

Blood Fungus/Mycosis Point

Test only on the left. To find the point, move toward the sternum in a straight line from the middle of the left collarbone. The location is in the third space between the ribs. For this point do not immediately paint the symbol on the body; rather you proceed as follows:

If the tensor shows a grade of 5 or higher, hold a card with 4 vertical lines on the test point and test it. A "balanced" reading here indicates a non-dangerous fungus and you do not have to do anything further. If the tensor still shows grade 3 or higher, however, draw 4 vertical lines on the point to energetically balance it. If you still test grade 5 or higher after this, you have to discover and remove the harmful blood fungus with the methods described in chapter 10.

Heavy Metal/Toxin Point (LI 19)

Test and balance only on the right side. The point is located below the nostril. Note that drawing on this point does not eradicate the heavy metal pollution, it simply establishes a temporary energetic balance. The toxic substances have to be removed in a special process (see chapter 11) in order for this process to be completed.

Allergy Point (SI 19)

Test and balance only on the right side. The point is found in front of the ear. As with the heavy metal point, balancing here does not eliminate the problem; it simply temporarily balances the body's energy. We note that an allergy still exists and that it will be tested and treated separately.

Retests

After the complete performance of the energy balance procedure, test again to see whether anything has improved/changed at the points you tested during the pre-test.

Spinal Reflexes on the Head

Proceed as described in the pre-test. If no improvement is shown, there could be a scar that has caused a field of disturbance—this could be an external scar or an internal one such as from a tooth extraction. Use your tensor to test the scars and see chapter 9 to learn how to clear the disturbance.

Testing the Spine

Also test the spine as described in the pre-test. In case the tensor still indicates pollution at any point, you can ask whether you should employ a sign on the spot (in the middle of the spine, left or right). If the answer is yes, test as to which sign from the energy circle is the correct one. Do not forget to ask how long this symbol should be left there.

Special Case: Y on the Body

We have already heard that the Ypsilon is a very valuable symbol that can energetically empower many things including food, medicines, or water. You can also place this symbol on the body to assist in processes in which the flushing of fluids is required, such as lymph blockages or edema. You must proceed very specifically and with the greatest care, however, or the body fluids might be further blocked and the patient will get worse. Before you use the Ypsilon on the body you must always test to see whether it should be inscribed upright or upsidedown.

This symbol can also be drawn on the right and left sides of the spine for intervertebral disc problems.

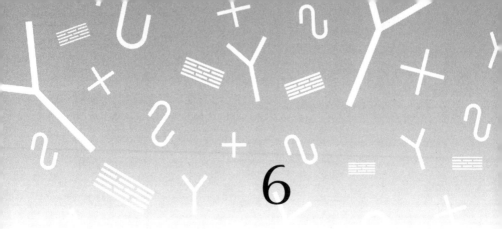

6

Storing and Clearing Healing Information

In addition to painting information directly on our bodies, it is often helpful to imprint more complex information onto something external, which can then be ingested or carried around for an extended period of time. The most common medium for imprinting and storing healing information is water, although there are many other effective media as well.

WATER

Water is the basis of all life. Our earth is covered with 70 percent water, a newborn baby consists of 75 percent water, and adults still hold around 60 percent of their body weight in water. The fluid that surrounds our cells (the extracellular matrix) contains over 90 percent water! Water saturates every cell of the body, absorbs and transmits warmth, and transports and exchanges the materials necessary to life, including sodium, potassium, calcium, magnesium, chloride, and phosphate. Across cellular membranes and connective

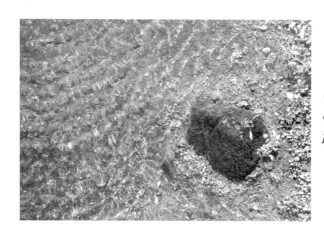

Our Earth is covered with 70 percent water.

tissues, water makes possible the communication between and among our cells.

Water is not only indispensable for our physical processes, however. It also influences all of our mental processes, our ability to concentrate and remember, and our emotional worlds.

From a chemical perspective, water (H_2O) is a combination of two hydrogen atoms and one oxygen atom (see figure below).

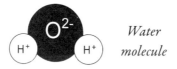

Water molecule

The next figure shows water molecules combined into a larger cluster of molecules connected by oxygen bridges.

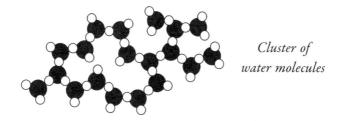

Cluster of water molecules

There are countless possibilities as to how oxygen bridges are formed. The latest findings of biophysics suggest that this ability of water to form clusters is partially due to the fact that water can store information. In the mid-1980s, Japanese scientist Masaru Emoto began to experiment with the energetic structure of water. Inspired by the American biochemist Dr. Lee H. Lorenzen, Emoto photographed crystals of frozen water under an electron microscope, and thereby discovered that water absorbs not only material substances but is also affected by thoughts, feelings, words, and images.

Emoto projected sound into samples of water (playing the music of Beethoven, Mozart, and various kinds of rock music), he "enchanted" the water by labeling it with words such as *love* or *hate*, and he observed and photographed the reaction of the water crystals to these inputs. The results were astonishing: To words or sentences associated with negative emotions (like the sentence, "You make me sick"), the crystals reacted with a disordered, chaotic structure—a lack of organization that brings to mind cancerous tumors or destruction. The water also reacted in this disordered way to heavy metal music.

By contrast, water labeled with words that arouse a positive association such as *love* or *thankfulness* formed wondrously beautiful crystals, as did the water samples bathed in the music of Mozart.

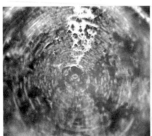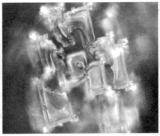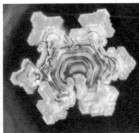

Pioneering photos by Japanese scientist Dr. Masaru Emoto: Water crystals were stimulated with the sound of heavy metal music (left) as well as the music of Elvis Presley (center) and Wolfgang Amadeus Mozart (right). But water also reacts to thoughts and emotions.

Apparently, water can absorb and respond to such messages. It reacts not only to information of a material sort but also to electromagnetic patterns of frequency and wavelength, such as are emitted from homeopathic medicines and Bach flower remedies, and even to tones, colors, thoughts, and emotions. Erich Körbler also used water as a "therapeutic substance"—a sort of messenger for transporting the vibration of healing symbols right into the cells of the body.

TRANSFERRING HEALING INFORMATION INTO WATER

Like Körbler, we can use water's ability to store information to transmit healing impulses. Viewed chemically, the water molecules remain unchanged during this informational process. Most probably, however, the informational content of the water crystals or the structure of the cluster is altered, which is what ultimately renders an influence wholesome or unwholesome.

For the transmission of healing information we use something called the "left-right effect." Regardless of which is your dominant hand, you hold the information you want to transfer in your left hand, and in your right hand you hold a glass of water or another object that you wish to imprint with healing information. For example, if you have tested negatively for milk, you can write the word "milk" on a piece of paper, along with the correct sign of reversal as determined by the energy circle (see chapter 4). Hold this piece of paper in your left hand while you hold a glass of water in your right hand. Then you visualize the information on the piece of paper flowing into the glass of water. When you drink the water, you absorb the healing impulse.*

---

*More information on this practice—including detailed examples—is included in chapter 10 of this book.

TRANSFERRING
HEALING INFORMATION
TO OTHER MEDIA

Pure water is the best medium for the transmission of healing information, because its power to store information, along with its extreme malleability, allow the desired information to make its way very quickly into every cell of the body. However, sometimes it is desirable to use another storage medium—one you can carry in your pocket, for example.

Stones

Precious and semiprecious stones—such as rock crystal, amethyst, and rose quartz—as well as metals like gold or silver—are good vehicles for transferring information. Many people know or sense intuitively what stones are good for them; if you are not sure, you should test the specific material. Sometimes even a favorite medium has a wavelength that is too strong or too weak for the specific work you wish to accomplish. In this case it is not very sensible to store additional information in it.

Once your selected medium has tested positive for the job at hand, you can begin the transmission of energy. The information transfer itself takes place exactly like the water transfer, that is, with the left-right effect. You hold the stone or metal in your right hand and the information you wish to transfer in your left hand, then visualize the transfer occurring. With a material object, you must then ask how you should use it: for example, whether you should carry it in a pocket or place it under your pillow, and for how long you should do so.

CASE STUDY

Tinnitus

Once I met a woman who was plagued by tinnitus, which had a lot to do with her stress at work. She had charged a small stone with information to effect a reversal in her psychological situation. She was supposed to carry the stone for two weeks. Shortly before the expiration of this time the stone fell on the floor in the bathroom and broke into countless pieces. Since the tinnitus also got much better, the stone was apparently sending a signal that its work was done . . .

Pieces of Jewelry

For pieces of jewelry the same thing is true as for stones. First ask whether the piece of jewelry is suitable for use in information transfer. Also you should ask whether a necklace should actually be worn around your neck, carried in a pocket, or whether perhaps it would be better to make use of a bracelet. This is because necklaces bring vibrational information to very sensitive areas—the thyroid and the hormonal system, and the thymus gland in the chest—so that the immune system can also be markedly influenced.

After the imprint is made, ask about the duration of time it should be used. Extending the healing symbol's work beyond this point can lead the information to reverse itself and become unwholesome for you.

Creams and Lotions

Healing creams and lotions provide a soothing way to apply healing information, especially in the case of skin outbreaks, or dry and irritated skin. First, find a simple cream that contains no unnecessary additives or perfumes—preferably from a shop that sells organic products—and test it for wholesomeness. If the base of the cream is good, you can transfer the desired information into it by means of the left-right effect. For example, you can write the word "itching" on a piece of paper, along with the sign of reversal that was indicated by your testing. You hold this piece of paper in your left hand, and a jar of cream in the right, then mentally transfer the information. You should also test here for how long it is sensible to use the cream.

Sugar Pellets

These little pellets—sometimes called "globules" or "blank homeopathic pellets"—can be purchased online from many homeopathic suppliers. As is done in homeopathy, information can be transferred to these small pills, which are ideal for children and other patients who prefer them.

Apples

These big, living, water-filled "blanks" are often used to transfer information when therapists apply New Homeopathy to horses. They can also, of course, be given to people. Be sure that the apple you choose tests well for wholesomeness before you imprint any information on it.

ERASING STORED INFORMATION

Just as information or vibrations can be imparted to various media, they can also be erased. With water transmissions erasure is not necessary, because you simply drink up all the water. When you rinse the glass out with warm water afterward, the information disappears.

Information that you have imprinted on an object like a stone or a bracelet, however, remains imprinted until you erase it again. The best time to do this is when the time span you previously determined for transmitting the healing information has passed. There are several effective methods of erasure discussed below.

Water

The simplest method is to hold the object under running water so that the imprinted information can flow off. It is nice to imagine Mother Earth gladly receiving the vibrations you no longer need.

Salt

Stones, metals, and pieces of jewelry can also be placed in good rock salt or crystal salt. It is important to inquire ahead of time whether this is suitable for your material, however, since salt can be harmful to some metals and stones. Also ask how long this energy cleansing process should last.

For materials that may be damaged by direct contact with salt, try this alternate method: Fill a large bowl with salt, and place a smaller bowl of plain water in the bowl of salt. Then place your stone or jewelry in the clear water for its cleansing. The salt can always be used again, but the water should be freshly replaced each time.

Sunshine

Rays of the sun have a great energetic vibratory power. They are best suited to charging things with new energy and for cleansing. For best results lay your material out in the sun on a linen cloth, inquire as to how long the process will take, and test again after this time period to see whether the imprinted information has been erased.

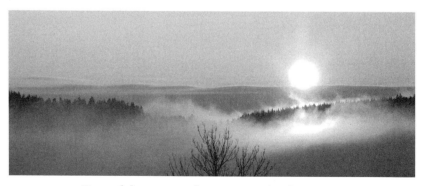

Rays of the sun can clear imprinted information.

Rituals

Simple rituals are also effective ways to remove unneeded information. For example, you can create a small shamanic ceremony, light incense, or say a simple prayer of thanks, like this one: *"Thank you, cosmic helpers, for giving me this healing information. I now ask Mother Earth to take on the information that is no longer needed. I thank you, Mother Earth."*

Overwrite with New Information

The simplest way to erase information that is no longer required is to imprint new information on top of it. In this case the previous information is simply "overwritten."

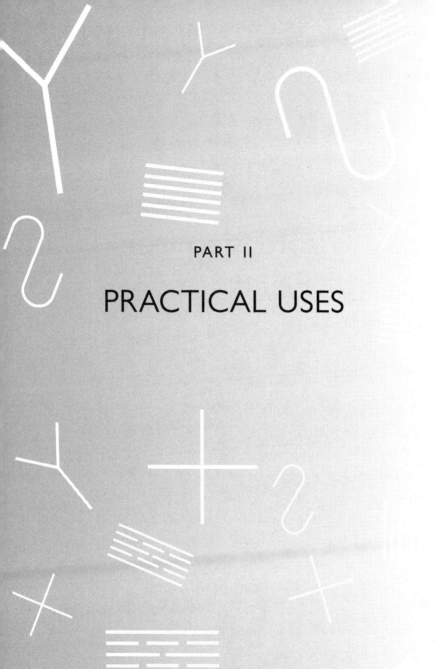

PART II

PRACTICAL USES

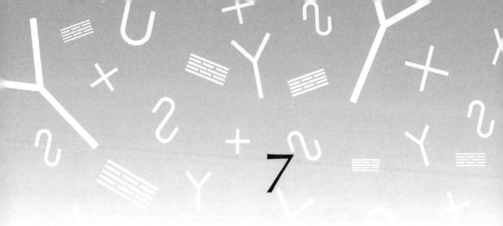

7

Protection from Electrosmog

Electrosmog is a general term for electrical fields of disturbance, which do not occur in nature and are made up of low- and high-frequency alternating fields. Only "non-ionizing" radiation, which has no radioactive effect, is counted as electrosmog, since radiation is already recognized as a health risk.

Although electrosmog cannot be seen or smelled, we know that it exists. It is a matter of controversy, however, whether or to what extent this radiation is harmful to humans. Magnetic or electromagnetic radiation under 1 milligauss (mG) is generally considered harmless. But if you consider that the electromagnetic charge in front of a computer carries 10–20 mG, and that this instrument is usually not the only one that surrounds us (or our children!) every day, then the issue becomes worrisome.

Moreover, the human organism consists in large part of water—an ideal conductor. Our bodily processes are governed by the rhythms and natural electrical impulses of lower frequencies. An intrusion into these natural processes by the technologizing of our environment leads undoubtedly to stress, and also can harm our organism and have incalculable effects on our health and well-being.

SENSITIVITY TO ELECTROSMOG

We know that some animals have special receptors that allow them to perceive magnetic and electromagnetic fields. Many fish navigate the sea with the help of magnetic fields, for instance, while pigeons and bats perceive the smallest alterations (measured in nanoteslas) in the Earth's magnetic field. The human nervous system, on the other hand, appears to react to electromagnetic influences without any special receptors. Since each person is a unique creation with very individual talents and sensibilities, the sensitivity to radiation can vary from person to person. Some will notice more clearly than others that a whole day under fluorescent lights, for example, exhausts the body and soul, or that a bad positioning of their beds can give them a sleepless night. In general, though, a healthy person will resist a negative radiation field longer than one already weakened by other illnesses.

Regardless of general effects, there are always people who are especially sensitive—those who perceive electrical, magnetic, or electromagnetic fields directly. Electrical sensitivity is different from an electrical allergy, in which the distribution of histamine proves a true allergic reaction. Electrical sensitivity can be partially evaluated by measuring the levels of melatonin produced by the pineal gland: laboratory experiments have shown that a pineal gland disturbed by electrosmog reduces its production of melatonin. Signs of insufficient melatonin levels include restlessness or a sleep disorder. As this proto-hormone is also a free-radical scavenger, insufficient levels can weaken the immune system and indirectly promote the genesis of cancer.

Increasing numbers of sensitive people report *hearing* electrical fields—whistling, knocking, buzzing, etc. Examples of complaints caused by electrical sensitivity are fever, redness, skin outbreaks, breathing difficulties, burning of the eyes, and light sensitivity. Over time, sufferers experience fatigue, decreased activity of all kinds, lack of concentration, sleep disorders, and nervousness. Some sensitive people who live close to transmitters for a long time can react to these fields with massive impairments, including confusion, extreme fatigue, and near-total disability.

CASE STUDY

Disturbed Sleep

Tomas Z. had always been a good sleeper. However, when he moved to a new house in 2003, he could not close his eyes all night. During the next two nights he also slept restlessly. I tested the position of his bed with the tensor and determined that there was a zone of disturbance in the head area. It was interesting to me that another experienced dowser who had already tested the rooms in the previous week was able to confirm these zones of disturbance. We therefore moved the bed, and the very next night the man was again able to sleep wonderfully—and has done so since.

TYPES OF ELECTROSMOG

In modern life, we are surrounded by dozens or hundreds of electrical fields everywhere we go. These fields fall into two major categories: electrostatic fields and low-frequency alternating fields.

Low-Frequency Electrical Alternating Fields

These fields originate from alternating voltage in electrical lines, switches, plugs, and all connected devices such as digital clocks, cell phones, computers, televisions, radios, and lamps, even when they are not turned on. These fields radiate outward from the devices in regular patterns and drop off as one moves farther away from the device in question.

Electrostatic Fields

Products made from synthetic materials have become more widespread in recent years. Artificial veneers with a wooden appearance, PVC, linoleum flooring, polyester curtains, synthetic carpets, and ubiquitous plastics provide a "charged" living space in their electrostatic interplay. Dry heated air also elevates the surface level electrical charge: many people know the small electrical shock they receive when they touch a door handle. Stress factors caused by electrostatic electricity can be reduced by the correct selection of building materials and furnishings.

MEASURING ELECTROSMOG WITH A TENSOR

A tensor can detect levels of electrosmog in the range of one nanometer. Simply test in the energy circle by putting the index finger of your non-dominant hand on the device you wish to test—on a radio, clock, plug, small appliance, or the electrical line in the wall, for example. If the tensor indicates grade 5 or higher, the frequency of this electromagnetic source is not wholesome for your organism and can sooner or later cause psychological, spiritual, or physical maladies. Satellite dishes or transmitters positioned outside the living space can be tested by pointing the palm of your hand in the direction of the instrument and directing your thoughts to the test object.

THE SYMBOL FOR
SUPPRESSING ELECTROSMOG

In the "pre-testing" section in chapter 5, we discussed how to test whether you are affected by electrosmog pollution: simply hold the tensor at the crown of your head (at the acupuncture point GV 20). If the tensor displays a circular movement (regardless of whether it is to the right or left) at the crown of the head, you have electrosmog pollution. This pollution can then be altered with the help of the Körbler symbol created for this purpose:

By looking at the electrosmog card for about two minutes, you will temporarily discharge the unwholesome radiation from your organism.

Moreover, the electrosmog symbol can be used to suppress the electrosmog disturbance from any small or large device, for example: alarm clocks, watches, television sets, computers, mobile phones, refrigerators, CD players, plugs, microwave ovens, lamps, and all devices made of metal, even those that are not attached to an electrical line. A simple way to use the electrosmog symbol is to make or buy stickers with the symbol printed on them. When you have tested an electrical device as being unwholesome for your organism, place a sticker on the device. Ask ahead of time where you should place the sticker, and whether you perhaps need a second or third one at another location on the device. Retest to see whether the symbol has balanced the unwholesome frequency, or at least improved it by a few degrees.

Of course, the electrosmog symbol cannot actually clean the radiation away; it is still present but has been made, in effect, more wholesome for your organism. This is an important step to take, especially when the source of the disturbance cannot simply be removed or changed, such as electrical outlets or lines in the wall.

The electrosmog symbol can also be enlarged on a piece of typing paper and laid under a computer or television. After a while, however, the paper itself can take on a charge, so it is important to retest every now and then to see whether the suppression of disturbance is still holding. Many practitioners have found that printing the symbol on a natural, uncolored cotton cloth helps it to last much longer.

FURTHER TIPS FOR AVOIDANCE OF ELECTROSMOG

The easiest way to prevent electrosmog pollution is to avoid it altogether: if you are already planning to move into a new apartment or house, you can act in a preventive way to lessen the unwanted low- or high-frequency radiation in your rooms.

- Avoid proximity to high-tension wires, overhead electrical lines, transformers, transmitters, and so forth.
- Electromagnetic radiation easily penetrates walls. Therefore consciously pay attention to what is under the bedroom. It is very unfavorable, for example, for the heater to be located there.
- Place your bed so that it is at least a meter (about two-and-a-half feet) away from any heating device.
- Avoid heaters in the floor.
- Turn off the television set and similar devices at night. Even the standby function (red light) should be turned off. Think about whether your children absolutely have to have a television or computer in their rooms.
- Sleeping directly under a halogen lamp with a transformer is approximately the same as lying under a high-tension wire.
- Do without clock radios, radios, and halogen lights, at least in your bedroom.

- Mechanical wristwatches and alarm clocks are more wholesome than quartz clocks.
- If you wear glasses, it is wise to test the material and shape of the frames before you buy them.
- Avoid having different metals mix in your mouth (e.g., simultaneously having fillings made of amalgam and gold), because this causes harmful alternating currents.

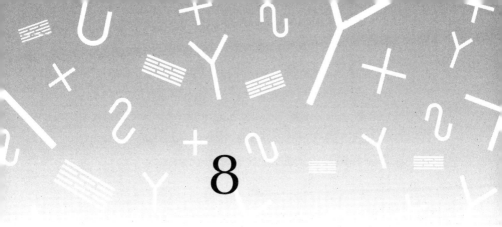

8

Harmonizing Geopathic Pollution

Geopathology (from the Greek: *ge,* meaning "earth," and *pathos,* meaning "sickness") is concerned with diseases that originate from extended exposure to polluted locations. Geopathic stresses generally arise from natural formations that are incompatible with one or more forces around them.

SOURCES OF GEOPATHIC STRESS

The most common zones of geopathic disturbance are formed by water veins, fault lines, or the electromagnetic grids that cover the Earth. While any single zone can be neutral or pathological, the greatest stress occurs where two or more of these zones overlap each other.

The Earth's Magnetic Field

The Earth's magnetic field is a naturally occurring field that extends in a north-south direction toward the poles. Its origins are still being investigated. All of life on Earth has adjusted itself to the Earth's magnetic field in the course of evolution and can live with it quite well. Some animals—migratory birds, sea turtles, and sharks, for example—even use the Earth's magnetic field to orient themselves. These natural fields are, as a rule, "balanced fields" that are in general wholesome for the organism.

Water Veins

Water veins are not actual veins but are substantial bodies of water in which there are currents and complex flowing movements. Rain trickles down into the ground, penetrates through many levels of rock, and forms subterranean watercourses wherever the stone cannot be penetrated. Where these watercourses come together, they form larger bodies of water or rivers that are constantly trying to move. These water veins can split into additional vertical and diagonal branches.

Such veins of flowing water can form zones of disturbance that generate pollution for living organisms. It is supposed that the negative energy is produced by the friction of the water against the hard surfaces surrounding it.

If a person sleeps for a long time over a water vein, she might gradually develop low levels of stress or tension, which can give rise

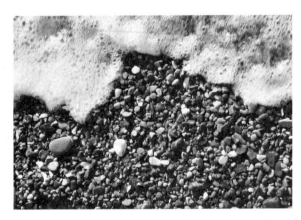

Flowing water can form zones of energetic disturbance.

to restless sleep, nightmares, headache, circulatory problems, and many other complaints. It is also possible that serious diseases, such as cancer or heart disorders, can arise after living for a long time over a water vein.

Grids

Grids are lines of friction that are joined together with the magnetic field of the Earth. In the past fifty years, a handful of researchers (such as Ernst Hartmann, M.D., and Manfred Curry, M.D., Siegfried Wittmann, and D. Francoir Peyre) have identified different grid systems with various alignments and various distances between their lines.

These grids are spread all over our planet in regular distances and still have not been thoroughly investigated. Reports and experimental results, however, show that as a rule they present zones of disturbance for living organisms and can lead to health-related difficulties.

The best known grids are:

- The Global Grid (Hartmann lines)
- The Diagonal Grid (Curry lines)
- Cubic Grid (Benker grid)

Some grids run with the cardinal directions (orthogonal grids), others run diagonally with respect to the cardinal directions (diagonal grids). Gridworks can have powerful effects on the human organism, especially when their lines cross one another. These crossing points amplify the harmful effect on our cells. These effects can be compared to those of water veins.

Global Gridwork (The Hartmann Grid)

The global gridwork that was discovered by Dr. Ernst Hartmann in the 1950s runs at intervals of about 2 meters in a north-south direction and at intervals of about 2.5 meters in an east-west direction. This grid is now generally recognized.

Hartmann was the first to be able to prove the connections between the gridlines and the occurrence of diseases. His work showed that healthy people have few problems when they sleep on top of a gridline, but lying on crossing-points causes sleep disturbances and, as laboratory experiments proved, can produce maladies of the most varied kinds.

Diagonal Grid (The Curry Grid)

The second radiation gridwork that spans the earth is named the Curry grid, after Dr. Manfred Curry. It runs diagonal to the Hartmann grid in the ordinal directions (between the cardinal points).

Unlike the Hartmann lines, the Curry grid is variable in its form and dependent, for example, on the phases of the moon. The intervals between the individual lines on the Curry grid run between 2.6 and 3.2 meters. Like the Hartmann lines, the Curry lines increase their damaging effects wherever they cross other lines or zones of disturbance.

The Cube Gridwork (Benker Cube System)

Anton Benker discovered another grid system in the 1960s—the Benker cube system. This grid can be conceived of as rectangular solids of 10 × 10 × 10 meters (approximately 33' × 33' × 33') lined up one after the other. The Benker cube system runs, like the Hartmann grid, in the north-south and east-west directions.

Rock Faults

Faults are subterranean fracture zones in the rock of the earth. They arise from movements underground, for example, when the tectonic plates of the earth rub against one another (in large instances, we know of this as an earthquake). Such fractures, cracks, splits, and sinkholes can have widths of several hundred meters.

According to Dr. Hartmann, fault lines are always pathogens, especially when they cross one another, water veins, or gridlines.

NEUTRALIZING GEOPATHIC POLLUTION

No expensive devices or special protective stickers are necessary to suppress geopathic pollution; our geometric forms are well suited to this purpose. The equilateral cross and the Jerusalem Cross are particularly effective at shielding us from a wide spectrum of disturbances caused by water veins, Hartmann or Curry lines, or intersections of these.

You may easily track down fields of disturbance beneath the earth and measure their wholesomeness/unwholesomeness with respect to the vibrations of your organism with the help of the tensor. For example, stand in front of your bed and point with your index finger to the place you want to inquire about. Think or say the words "disturbance zone," "water vein," "cross-point," and so forth, and observe the degree indicated by the tensor.

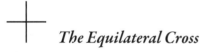

The Equilateral Cross

If your tensor indicates an unwholesome condition, place the equilateral cross under the bed and retest. This symbol made of two equally long strokes has been used since ancient times in different cultures as a protective sign.

In many cases this symbol brings balance right away or can at least make the place of disturbance a few degrees more wholesome for your organism.

The Jerusalem Cross

In some cases the simple cross is insufficient for the suppression of the disturbance, and the Jerusalem Cross is better suited. Therefore, test for pollution by water veins, cross-points, and so on, with this symbol as well. Possibly the best results are brought about by a combination of the equilateral cross and the Jerusalem Cross. Always inquire as to where the symbol should be placed—perhaps under your head, under the foot of the bed, or in the middle.

The Y Symbol

The third possibility for harmonizing geopathic pollution consists of the use of the Ypsilon symbol. This, too, can convert unwholesome energies of the earth into wholesome ones for your organism. Nature itself demonstrates this tactic: The trunks of trees that grow over water veins will split in two, in order to ameliorate the negative energy. The trees thereafter grow in the form of a Y.

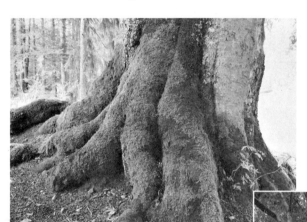

Notice the Y shape in nature, shown here in tree roots and trunks.

9

Clearing Disturbances
Caused by Scars

In the modern practice of medicine, scars that form after injuries or surgery have little more significance than to show evidence of healing. They are important to the practice of energy medicine, however, because scars very often create fields of disturbance. This is true not only for especially large, sensitive, painful, or weather-sensitive scars, but also for small inconspicuous ones, which can nonetheless be associated with an experience causing a blockage. Even internal scars, such as those caused by abdominal surgeries, tonsillectomies, tooth extractions, or episiotomies can test negatively.

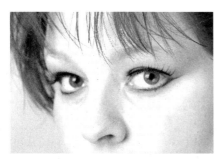

Scars very often form fields of disturbance, including forgotten, internal scars—for instance, those formed after a tooth extraction or an episiotomy.

The hard, inflexible scar tissue blocks the streams of energy that flow in the meridians, thereby affecting all the organs and other zones these meridians are supposed to supply with energy. A field of disturbance linked to a scar can cause large and small problems, including health disorders and chronic diseases.

Besides the more-or-less well-known methods of scar work, such as the injection of fluids beneath the scars in neural therapy or "scratch" therapy (cruciform scratching over the surface of the scar with a sharp object, e.g., a dental tool), we can also use healing symbols in a simple and painless way to neutralize scar tissue problems.

EXTERNAL SCARS

Test the scar as usual with the tensor and wait for the result. You can also simply touch the area with your fingertip or go along the length of a longer scar with your index finger.

When treating an external scar, we use only a 1-line symbol or a sine curve, not the full range of signs of the energy circle. If a scar tests negatively, hold a card with one line on it over the scar (as if you were striking through the scar with the line) and then retest. If you get a balanced reading at that point (grade 1), then paint the line directly on the scar so that the vibration will be completely harmonized. If the line is not sufficient to attain grade 1, hold a sine curve card on the scar and observe the reading again. If it's back to grade 1, paint the sine curve in the direction of the scar. With longer scars it may be necessary to draw several individual lines on different tested areas.

INTERNAL AND
HARD-TO-REACH SCARS

Internal or hard-to-reach scars are tested in the energy circle by simply asking about them, for example, "Does this episiotomy scar need to be treated?" Results above grade 5 are harmonized with water transference using the standard energy circle signs. (See the following chapter for more detailed instructions about water transference methods.)

CASE STUDY

Thyroid Nodules and Large Burn Scar on the Neck

Ms. H., forty years of age, had had a strawberry birthmark removed from her neck/breast area at one year of age, after which she was accidentally left under a radiation device. Since then she had had an approximately 15 x 15 cm-size burn scar with a thick swelling, which she suffered from especially during puberty. Because of this thick scar, she could not bend her head backward. She also had problems with her parents.

Ms. H. had recently visited a doctor for painful hemorrhoids, and was told they would need to be surgically removed. In addition, she had a history of thyroid nodules and fluctuation levels of thyroid hormones, which had not been successfully controlled by thyroid medicine.

Treating this long-standing scar required a range of methods. During the course of several sessions, we drew signs directly on the scar and used water transfers to impart additional information. We also used the detoxification protocol as described in chapter 11, homeopathic remedies, and psycho-meridian information as described in chapter 12.

Ms. H. made several appointments for treatment. In the beginning I stabilized her through an energy balance and freed the scar on her neck by using drawn signs and a water transfer with the words: "Scar Breast" and the symbol ‖⌒∪.

Her psycho-meridian indicated a problem with her father. We wrote "relationship to father" on a piece of paper with a sign on it, which she was to look at often. Additionally, I prescribed a homeopathic medicine for her that I had previously tested.

At the next retesting her energy-balance status had changed for the better and the large scar had improved by two gradations. Due to the amalgam poisoning that was indicated on the meridian points during the energy balance, I now performed a mercury drain-off for the patient and tested her for the precise dose of chlorella algae, a liver medicine, and goldenrod for her kidneys. Additionally, she received the tree-essence of oak stalk.

A little while later the healing reactions set in, which Ms. H. reported to me on the telephone. The first reaction was that the hemorrhoids, which were supposed to have been removed by surgery, had disappeared. Two weeks later the scar on her neck burst open and bled with a thin fluid. At the places where the bleeding stopped, new pink baby skin appeared. Ms. H. was able for the first time since puberty to bend her head back again without pain and a pulling sensation.

For a while the patient sweated at night, her eyes were swollen, and she had the feeling that the neck was getting thicker, though she no longer had any nodules. She coughed at night and felt that this was due to the blood pressure pills she took. Psychologically Ms. H felt very good. She noticed that these varied symptoms started to get better when she took the medicine for draining off the amalgam.

After the time period for taking the medicines for draining off the amalgam had elapsed, we retested; two of these medicines were to be continued. We discontinued the blood pressure pills with a slow and gradual replacement by water transfer.

A month later Ms. H. had a check-up examination by her doctor: her thyroid values were completely normal and the nodes had disappeared. She was very thankful.

10

Rewriting
Chronic Conditions
with Water Transmission

Erich Körbler conducted many experiments with information transfer into water and into other media, and frequently presented his results to the public in clear, easy-to-understand terms. He found that the coupling of line-sine curve combinations with the power of water makes it possible to "rewrite" information that has led to chronic symptoms. Whether the problematic vibrations have come to us from the outside (e.g., from pollen or environmental pollution) or from within (emotions, thoughts), we know that a recurring problem means the affected cells have been storing unhealthy information and producing new cells according to a faulty matrix. The cells need to be reminded of their original healthy pattern, which is best done by drinking water that has been imprinted with the desired new information. This process "erases" or rewrites the old, unwholesome information, transforming it into wholesome information. The signs that we especially want to use here are sine curve, 1-line sine curve, and 2-line sine curve.

With this method negative influences or unwholesome vibrations that create conditions such as allergies, food aversions, harmful fungal blood infections, or toxicity from mercury can be rewritten and drained away. Even entrenched dogmatic beliefs and patterns of behavior can receive a healing impulse from water transfer.

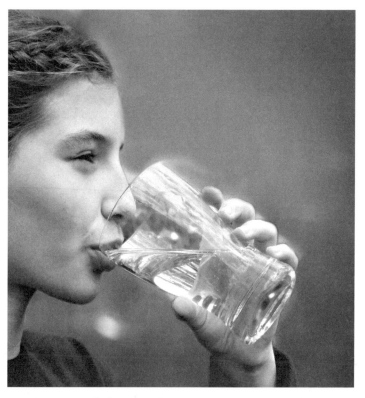

By storing wholesome information in water, we can erase unwholesome information in the body.

INSTRUCTIONS FOR PERFORMING A WATER TRANSFER

For the following example imagine that you have determined a hazel pollen allergy in the energy circle at grade 6.

1. Hold the information that is to be transferred into the water in your left hand. In this case you would be holding a piece of paper on which you have written "hazel pollen" and drawn ∏ᴜ (the symbol for grade 6) over it with a thick marker.

2. Hold a glass filled with water in your right hand. The glass must be real glass rather than plastic and should have no words or images on it. The water should be as pure and as free of carbonation as possible.

3. Now pay attention to the information you want to transfer: Imagine that the information is flowing through your body from left to right in the direction of the glass of water. Remain completely relaxed, and do not over concentrate. The left hand absorbs energy from the paper, and the right hand projects it into the water.

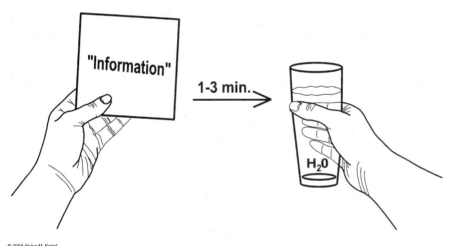

Transferring information to water

Information is received through the eye, the sensory nerve cells, and the chakra (energetic point) on the palm of the hand, and is projected into the water via the same routes. After three minutes you can be certain that the transfer has been concluded and the water has absorbed sufficient information. Now drink the water at your own pace, and the information will be passed to the cells of your body. With this "left-to-right method" you can transfer one-to-one any information that gives your organism a positive impulse. As we saw in chapter 6, these transferences can also be accomplished with other materials like stones or colors.

DETERMINING THE LENGTH OF TREATMENT

Next ask how often you should repeat this water transfer, because a stable condition can only be achieved by repetition of the water transfer. You might begin by asking "Should this medicine be taken for one day?" Assuming your tensor indicates "yes" move on to asking about two days, then three days, and so on, until you get a "no." If it seems that it is going to be weeks rather than days, ask "Should this medicine be taken for weeks?" Then ask if it should be one week, two weeks, or three weeks, and so on, until you get a "no." This same step-up process can be used to determine the appropriate number of doses per day.

TREATING ALLERGIES

Allergies and food intolerances often respond quite well to information encoded into water. The unwholesome information that leads to the habitual allergic response can be overwritten with the correct symbol of reversal to create a new, non-allergic response. If you suspect a lactose intolerance, for instance, because you react to milk products with a stomachache or diarrhea, you would proceed as follows.

Making use of the energy circle, ask: "How do I tolerate milk?" Wait for the indication. We will assume you get an indication with the tensor of grade 7, that is, a leftward turning circle. Now write the word "milk" on a piece of paper and draw the harmonizing symbol for grade 7 over it with a heavy marker. Next, take a glass of water in your right hand.

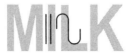

Hold the piece of paper in your left hand and look at it. Imagine how the information flows through your body into the water and is absorbed by the water. This process lasts about three minutes. The information transfer is then complete. Drink the water at your own pace.

Next ask how long this medicine should be taken, as described in "Determining the Length of Treatment" on the facing page.

CASE STUDY

Atopic Eczema

Shortly before Christmas 2005 Ms. L. came to my office completely unnerved. The holidays were just ahead, and she was very worried that she would be completely at the mercy of the itchy skin on her lower left leg. The itching plagued her constantly, especially at night in her warm bed. She reported that the eczema had been going on for years and always got worse in the fall, with swelling and reddening of her lower legs. The examination in my husband's office (he is a general practitioner) resulted in a diagnosis of atopic eczema with venous congestion and swelling. The energy diagnosis showed severe blockage at various meridian points and several conspicuous liver points. Some toxin and allergy points were also indicated.

During the spine testing (see page 57 in chapter 5), lumbar vertebrae 1, 2, and 3 were indicated. In connection with this the patient complained of sciatic nerve pain that recurred continually. She had visited several doctors recently, but without any improvement.

Testing for the main allergens revealed that rye, wheat, and eggs were particularly problematic. Nuts, oranges, nickel, and some pollens also reacted. Additionally, the patient tested positive for a few types of mold.

From December of 2005 to May of 2006, treatment with the bar codes and some supplements eliminated the most conspicuous allergies; within a few weeks the itching disappeared, as well as other minor allergy symptoms. The patient continued to avoid rye and wheat, but was able to reintegrate all the other foods back into her diet. Above all, she was able to wear a silver-nickel necklace, which she had been completely unable to do before her treatment. She lost nearly 18 pounds, and her legs grew smooth and lost their redness. Finally, the mold sensitivity also disappeared. The healing succeeded so quickly thanks to Ms. L.'s disciplined and conscientious behavior. She was willing and able to make changes in her diet and habits and thus fully embraced her healing.

When using water transfers to alleviate allergies, food intolerances, heavy metal pollution, or even psychological concerns, the degree of the pollution has to be brought down step by step. This means that a water transfer with 2-line sine curve or 1-line sine curve usually has to be followed by other operations on the same subject with the next lower symbol.

Therefore, inquire at the conclusion of the first transfer (e.g., 2-line-sine curve) whether another symbol is necessary (e.g., 1-line sine curve) in order to balance the intolerance. Now ask again about the duration of the water transfer. Experience shows that after the transfers for a particular theme have been stepped down to a sine curve, the desired vibratory balance is produced.

CASE STUDY

Attention Deficit Disorder

Robert, born in 1993, was a miracle child. During his gestation his mother had had two infections and experienced premature labor. The child slept only about three to four hours at night and an additional one to two hours during the day. His physical development was somewhat delayed, and he had a club foot. At six months the baby fell over a rock step and went to sleep immediately, but showed no peculiarities after the fall.

Upon entering preschool at 3¾ years of age, Robert suffered separation anxiety and cried a lot when he was separated from his mother. Entering school at 6¾ years was also difficult: Robert was interested in anything but school. In the fall of 2001 Robert developed breathing difficulties at night. A thorough housecleaning was done as a result, and Robert was started on medicines containing cortisone to control his asthma. In 2002/2003 a test confirmed Attention Deficit Disorder Syndrome, and the boy received a half tablet of the active ingredient Ritalin twice daily. During vacations the medicine was discontinued. When this dosage did not achieve the desired results, Robert's dose was increased to a half tablet three times daily, seven days a week. Since beginning the medicine the boy no longer had asthma. He regularly received osteopathic treatments as well.

In April of 2004 Robert's mother brought him to my office. We initially did the energy balance and worked on the difficult weaning and separation from his mother with water transfers. I tested that we could replace the Ritalin for two days a week over the coming five weeks. This was done by transferring the information

"Ritalin," along with the correctly tested bar codes, to sugar pellets and water. Two homeopathic medicines additionally tested well and were administered to the patient.

At the next appointment testing revealed that Ritalin could be replaced in the manner mentioned above for three days each week. When I did the energy balance again, it indicated heavy metal toxicity, so I began a heavy metal drain-off.* The concept "ADD-Child-Robert" tested with a great disturbance and was drained off using the water transfer.

After this things went well for Robert. His mother reported that he felt better than when he was on Ritalin. He was very motivated to do everything correctly, complied correctly with his directions, and demonstrated no peculiarities.

In August of 2004 I spoke again with Robert's mother. Things continued to go well for him, his grades were in the middle range, he had not gotten worse academically, and we were able to replace Ritalin on additional days.

In the middle of September, testing showed that now the sixth and seventh day of taking the medicine Ritalin could be replaced by information transfer. Robert now took medicinal information exclusively in the form of informed water and sugar pellets. Things were going excellently for him, and the nausea and stomach pains he had constantly suffered from while he was taking Ritalin had disappeared completely.

Finally we conducted an allergy test and found disturbances associated with wheat germ oil, benzoate, calcium phosphate, and aluminum. We drained these off by means of water transfers.

It should also be noted that aluminum makes one restless, causes concentration disturbances, and generally causes symptoms similar to Alzheimer's. In my opinion this constellation of symptoms is

---

*See chapter 11 for more information about this process.

labeled "Alzheimer's" among adults and Attention Deficit Disorder among children. To our great joy things continue to go well for Robert.

"Y" FOR STABILIZATION AFTER REWRITING

It is important that you repeat the water transfer as often and regularly as indicated by the tensor readings so that a stable condition can be achieved. After the time span of the transfer, and whatever stepping-down has been indicated, the tensor will indicate "okay" with grade 1. Now use the symbol "Y" to stabilize this balanced condition, virtually as a signal meaning: "It's good now." To stick with our "milk" example from above, you will now write the word "milk" one last time on a piece of paper. Draw a large Y over it and do the water transfer again. Test again as to how often you should repeat this process (usually one to two days). Only then is the drain-off process for "lactose intolerance" complete.

The time span for drinking the informed healing water as indicated by testing can vary tremendously, from "a few days" to "daily several times" over weeks. The entire time span for the process is best written out like a prescription on a piece of paper. For example:

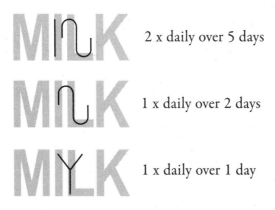

MILK   2 x daily over 5 days

MILK   1 x daily over 2 days

MILK   1 x daily over 1 day

CASE STUDY

Sinusitis

Klara was sixty-one years old, married, and had a twenty-two-year-old daughter. For the past few years she had been living in a small house in the country, most months apart from her family. A "nervous intestine" with a tendency toward diarrhea had been with her since her kindergarten days. In her adult years allergies triggered by hazelnut, birch, and ragweed caused typical symptoms in the eyes and nose and then led to asthma. About ten years previously, she'd been diagnosed with a yeast infection of the intestine and went through a cleansing program to clear it. Her gallbladder was surgically removed in 1973 because of gall stones. A few foods, such as milk, celery, stone fruit, hazelnuts, and cabbage, were not well tolerated. Pseudo-allergic reactions resulted especially when exposed to food additives, dyes, paints, and cleaning materials. The symptoms resulted in sinusitis, bronchitis, skin outbreaks, conjunctivitis, and accompanying exhaustion and fatigue.

Now Klara came to my office exhausted and with an acute case of sinusitis. At the beginning of her treatment we did the energy balance. Especially conspicuous in the testing were the points of the large intestine and liver: they were subsequently painted with the corresponding bar code in the green color indicated by some additional testing. A conversation about the possible causes of her symptoms gave reason to suppose that the smell of paint from having the ceiling in her workshop painted was involved. This was confirmed in testing: "ceiling paint, workshop," which tested with a strong disturbance. I tested for the dose and duration of the water transfer and told Klara how to continue performing the water transfers at home.

At first Klara did not believe in her ability to transfer information into water or that this method would work very quickly for her.

So she did not immediately begin the therapy. A day later, however, she had a dream in which she remembered: "I should write an essay about the meaning of water in a dream. I hesitated, I did not think I could do it, but my teacher encouraged me. I wrote how important water is for us humans and that the earth is called the blue planet because it consists of such enormous surfaces of water. Water carries ships, conducts energy; water helps to bring blood into each of our cells. We can live awhile without food, but not without water and air."

The next morning Klara began a successful course of water transfer. Her symptoms improved dramatically in six days, and by the conclusion of the treatment they had completely disappeared.

IMPORTANT: NOT TOO MUCH AT ONE TIME!

We recommend that you transfer no more than two to three pieces of information into water at one time. The bioenergetic system needs time to reduce blockages gradually, and too much can overload it. Inquire with the tensor in cases where you have any doubt.

Even when the process is simple, and only one repetition of a water transfer actually succeeds in eliminating the problem, reversals can occur further on down the line. In such cases we assume that there are other issues complicating the person's healing, and might continue by investigating the psycho-meridian or chakra balance as described in chapters 12 and 13.

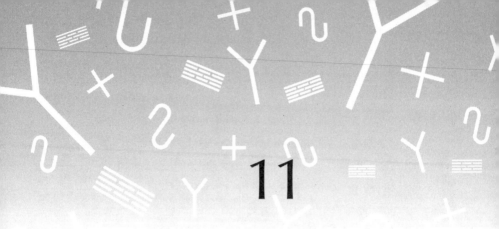

11

Detoxification

The methods of informational medicine are particularly well suited to supporting the body in removing and eliminating toxins. If the toxin point (Large Intestine 19 under the right nostril) tests negatively during the energy balance, it is then painted with the appropriate sign of reversal on the spot as first aid. While this procedure will temporarily balance the body's energies, the toxins themselves still remain and need to be treated more specifically.

As a follow-up the therapist can ascertain the specific environmental toxins that are causing harm by means of test lists or special heavy metal testing sets. Toxins can be materials from living spaces, exhaust gases, dyes, vaccines, narcotics, medicines, and so forth. After this testing the patient will know which materials to avoid in the future, and the process of elimination can begin.

Along with aluminum, cadmium, nitrates, and formaldehyde, just to name a few environmental toxins, there are very frequently health problems associated with the heavy metal amalgam, which is still used as material for filling teeth. Along with silver, amalgam contains amounts of copper, tin, and about 50 percent mercury. Mercury is also introduced into the body via certain vaccines, as well as from air, water, and some foods (many fish, for example, contain high levels of mercury).

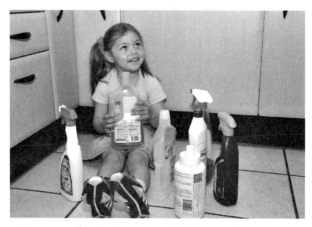

Be aware of polluting materials in your living spaces.

In the United States dental amalgam is considered a medical device and is regulated by the Food and Drug Administration (FDA). The FDA considers amalgam fillings safe for adults and children ages six and above. However, it is fact that people who have several different metals as tooth fillings (e.g., gold alloys, amalgam, silver) demonstrate elevated levels of mercury, and mercury is a known neurotoxin. Mercury in dental fillings can be dissolved by electrolysis in the mouth and thereby enter the body, where it is generally stored in fat tissue. Because nerve tissue is surrounded by fat (the brain consists of up to 60 percent fat tissue), much of these toxins get into the brain and nerves. Mercury can also build up in organs and lead to various disorders and diseases, including food allergies and increased susceptibility to fungal infections in the blood and intestines.

PURIFICATION AND DETOXIFICATION AS THE "MOTHER OF ALL THERAPIES"

When performing an energy balance for someone, you will often find amalgam toxicity occurring along with some allergies or food sensitivities. In these cases it is best to follow the steps for amalgam elimination first as described below; the allergy symptoms will often improve by this measure alone. In fact many symptoms are actually caused by underlying metal toxicity, so following the detoxification procedures can alleviate many ailments at one time. This is why detoxification is sometimes referred to as the "mother of all therapies."

Unlike some other toxins, amalgam and mercury can be removed from the body in a bound form. That is, certain molecules will bind to the mercury molecules in the body, forming water-soluble complexes that are ultimately excreted in urine or stool. Standard medicine uses the compounds DMPS and DMSA for this purpose, while natural medicine practitioners often turn to chlorella algae to accomplish these same ends.

In New Homeopathy we also make use of chlorella, a freshwater algae, along with other herbal medicines that support the body in its detoxification processes. Herbs such as goldenrod, bear's garlic, and certain bitters are especially helpful for the liver and kidneys, which are primarily responsible for this kind of detoxification. Several companies offer special test sets that include effective drainage agents. It is important to do research—over the Internet, directly with the companies, or with your doctor or healing practitioner. Together, the combination of New Homeopathy symbols and targeted herbal support has shown to be an effective way to drain mercury/amalgam contamination from the body.

DRAINING HEAVY METALS IN PRACTICE

Over time you can drain mercury or other toxins by following the steps below. In this example we are clearing mercury pollution, but you could as easily substitute the word "amalgam" or "aluminum" or whatever poison you are trying to drain.

1. Use the tensor and the energy circle to test how severe the poisoning is. Have you or your patient say the word "mercury" and see how the tensor responds.

2. If your tensor shows a grade 5 or above, write the word "mercury" on a piece of paper and paint the corresponding sign of reversal over it. (The correct sign of reversal will be the one associated with the grade indicated by your tensor in the energy circle.)

3. Follow the water transfer instructions provided in the previous chapter, determine the length of treatment, and remember to finish your treatment with the stabilizing force of the Ypsilon (see pages 94–103).

4. Test for which herbal medicines you should incorporate into your detoxification treatment:

   • Chlorella algae: How much, how long? A range of 5 to 100 pieces daily is certainly possible and frequently necessary for individual dosages in order to be able to bind to the poisons freed by the symbols.
   • Agents for drainage of the kidneys (e.g., solidago/goldenrod): How many drops, how often (one or two times daily), how long?
   • Agents for drainage of the liver (e.g., dandelion, rosemary): How much, how often, how long?

In practice, after you perform the draining of amalgam or other toxins in this way, you may notice an "onionskin" effect—that is, further toxic pollutions that were previously hidden may now show up in your testing. These can then be drained off step by step with the help of healing symbols and drainage agents.

CASE STUDY

Hay Fever

I had successfully treated Peter T. (born 1961) in the past for severe allergies. Now he came to my office after a two-year hiatus because his allergies had returned. During the energy balance I ascertained amalgam and mercury toxicity. Upon inquiry the patient said that twelve years previously he had had six amalgam fillings removed without having a drain-off done. This amalgam toxicity had not been indicated in our work two years earlier, most likely because the amalgam was at that time still encapsulated in the cells and not yet detectable via testing.

The amalgam drainage for Peter consisted of transferring to water the information "amalgam, mercury" with the signs that had been tested out. After about three weeks the tensor no longer detected amalgam in the connective tissue, so we began to draw out the hidden reserves of it using cilantro extract. By adding cilantro or cilantro extract to food, intercellular amalgam can be mobilized out of the nervous system, at which point it can be detected and drained with the tensor and healing symbols. We detected and drained aluminum at the same time, which led to stomach complaints and headaches for a short period. After a few weeks, however, Peter felt considerably better.

At this point, yet more toxins were indicated—polio and tetanus, caused by earlier vaccines. We drained that, treated the psychic pollution of Peter's first hay fever attack thirty years before, and rewrote his existing allergies altogether: oak, birch, rose, broom, snapdragon, and zinnia. In mid-August 2004 all allergies with their attendant symptoms disappeared. I released the patient free of complaints.

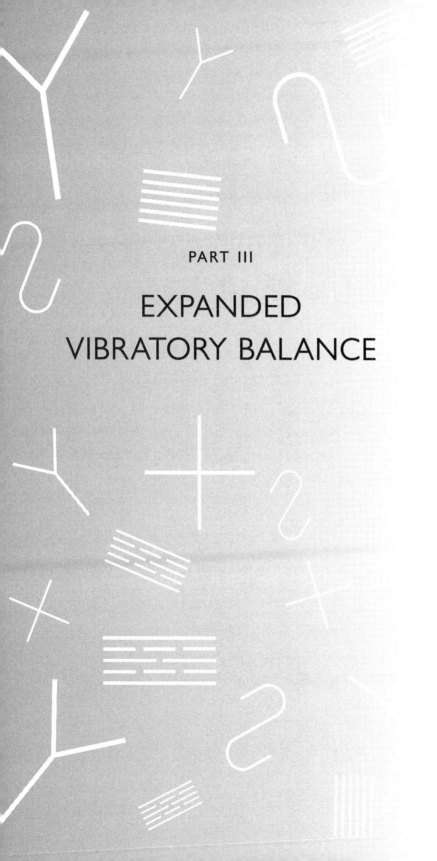

PART III

EXPANDED
VIBRATORY BALANCE

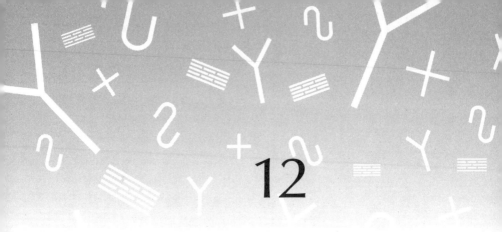

12

Working with the Psycho-Meridian

The psycho-meridian is a timeline used to trace the point of origin of a particular psychological blockage. For many therapists practicing New Homeopathy, work with the psycho-meridian counts as one of the most important aspects of the healing process, because many diseases or disturbances can have underlying psychological causes that are otherwise very difficult to detect. If a particular disturbance does not rebalance after you have tried many ways to clear it (scar clearing, detoxification, etc.), it may be an indication that there is an unresolved psychological conflict that has its origin in a past event in the person's life.

Along the psycho-meridian, which runs from the first vertebra of the neck along the midline of the skull to the crown of the head, the time period and theme of long-standing blockages can be tested for in wonderful ways. The psycho-meridian represents a sort of "lifeline" that the therapist tests with the tensor, beginning (at the present) at the top of the skull, and moving backward down to the neck vertebra, which represents the point of birth. By tracing a non-dominant finger down this lifeline, we can see by where the tensor reacts when in a person's life any particular disturbance began. In treatment the blockages that are closest to the present are always worked on first. Once this process is complete you can go back further into the past.

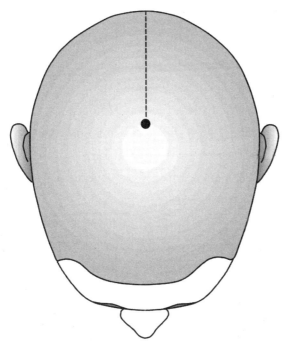

The psycho-meridian

TESTING THE PSYCHO-MERIDIAN

1. With your non-dominant index finger, point at GV 20 at the highest point on the head, and slowly move your finger in the direction of the first vertebra of the neck (the indentation upon which the head sits). During this think about the theme you wish to inquire about.

2. Observe the reading of the tensor you are holding in your other hand. Stop at the point at which the tensor first registers

a negative reading and estimate the age. If the patient is, for example, forty-four years old and you get a reading of grade 5 at approximately the middle of the line, the disturbance occurred at twenty-two years of age. If this occurs, ask the patient if something significant happened to him at that age. His reaction can be accompanied by (often strong) emotions. Therefore, this work should remain reserved for experienced therapists or be conducted during a seminar.

In working with the psycho-meridian the therapist should always give the patient the opportunity to remain discreet: He does not have to tell the person giving the treatment what life experience lies behind the disturbance. It is much more important that the patient himself gets emotional access to the event causing the inner conflict.

3. It may prove helpful to test which emotions this event is connected to. New Homeopathy relies on the classification system of the Chinese five element system, in which an element is ascribed to each major emotion such as rage, aggression, sadness, and so on. Special charts exist that, in connection with dowsing, can help to reveal these emotions. For those who don't have access to a chart, you can simply write down or say aloud the name of an emotion that is suspected and use your tensor to determine if it is related to the trauma.

TREATING THE PSYCHO-MERIDIAN

After testing on the psycho-meridian has helped to reveal the age, event, and specific emotions connected to a particular disturbance, the symbols of balance are once more brought into play. Then, for example, the following information can be written on a piece of paper: "22 years old, abortion, loss, pain." The appropriate grade is then painted on it with a heavy marker, and this information is used to create healing water for the patient. As described in the chapter on water transfers, the individual steps and the whole span of time for the harmonizing of the vibrations are then determined through testing. (See chapter 10.)

CASE STUDY

Fear and Panic Attacks

In March of 2005 Shakti came to my office to heal her panic attacks. Born in 1974, she was now a refined and delicate young woman and a physical therapist by profession. She had suffered from panic attacks since she was six years old. At the age of twelve she did not dare leave the house for a whole year because of her anxiety. Later, she was several times a victim of sexual abuse. Shakti was afraid to eat food that had a shell or peeling, she was afraid to fly, and she was fearful of water. She also complained of congestion, food intolerances, and allergies.

Fears are often somaticized so that people develop physical symptoms that only indirectly have anything to do with the body. The way out of these symptoms is to first heal the fear, then focus later on the questions of physical health (drainage of heavy metals, food intolerances, etc.).

With the help of the energy balance I tested for the location of the imbalance in Shakti's energy system and painted the appropriate meridian points with geometric symbols. After this, I used the psycho-meridian to ascertain the age at which Shakti's trauma really began.

The tensor indicated a problem in the second year of life. Shakti could not remember what had happened at that time, but together we were able to discover what basic emotions were tied to this event. The discovery and acceptance of the underlying emotions proves to be good at helping us to get closer to a trauma, especially when the incident causing them has been repressed or forgotten.

We discovered rage, rejection, and panic. We worked together on the rewriting of the trauma with a water transfer, which Shakti employed in the following weeks. I also showed her how she could consciously perceive her fears whenever they arose. I recommended to her that she allow them to arise and even embrace and welcome them. As a support for the healing process we imprinted tones and colors (blue) on a rose quartz stone that Shakti carried wrapped up in a cloth and tied around her ankle. It was her idea to wear the stone on her person this way; I usually recommend the pants pocket.

Two months later Shakti came to my office. Her whole being had been positively transformed. She reported to me that her panic attacks had completely disappeared and the problem in her relationship had been resolved. Given Shakti's difficult past these changes seemed like a miracle to her, for which both of us were thankful. Now that the pressing psychological problems had been resolved, we continued to work together on the purification of her cells and her physical health. By means of rewriting into water, we drained off heavy metals and treated her food intolerances.

Shakti felt better than ever, both physically and psychologically, and now looked forward to life with confidence. Her case is a good example of the wonderful possibilities of this method to help people psychologically as well as physically.

The geometric signs work naturally with physical, emotional, and psychic problems. Through information reversal the disturbed energy that caused the blockage and perhaps manifested disease is transformed into something harmonious. Energy that flows freely and unhindered stimulates the powers of the body to heal itself. In this way psychologically manifested illnesses can also experience healing. Many patients describe the work on the psycho-meridian as a breakthrough session, because they experience an initial jump start in the process of recovery.

Work with the psycho-meridian has especially proven itself in connection with unresolved psychological conflicts, psychological blockages, addictions, traumas, anxieties, and phobias.

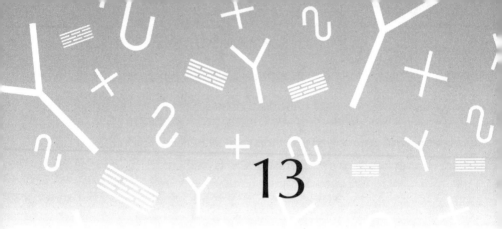

13

Chakra Balance

In addition to the psycho-meridian, chakra and aura therapy offers manifold possibilities for removing the causes of physical and psychological disorders.

THE CHAKRAS

Chakras are energy centers that absorb information from the morphic field through various levels of the aura. Chakras conduct this information into the meridians, process it, and then emit it again. There are seven main chakras or power centers along the midline of the body, each of which has a different area of function, and numerous smaller chakras that are spread throughout the body.

The Root Chakra
The root chakra lies between the sacrum and the coccyx and constitutes our connection to the earth. Here, life energy is absorbed and conducted to the other chakras. People with a well-developed root chakra are full of life, radiate brightness, and usually have no problems materially. If the root chakra is blocked, there is often a lack of

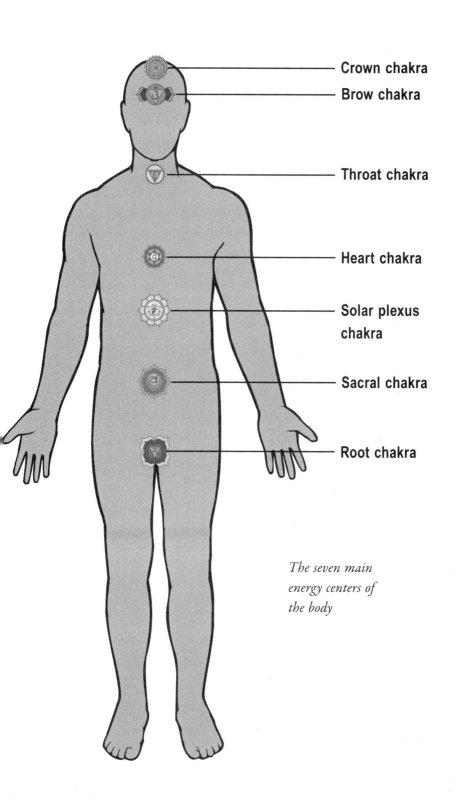

Crown chakra

Brow chakra

Throat chakra

Heart chakra

Solar plexus
chakra

Sacral chakra

Root chakra

*The seven main
energy centers of
the body*

vital power and the whole organism is not well supplied with energy.

The Sacral Chakra

The sacral chakra is situated below the navel. Its themes are sensuality, desire, and abandon, which refer not just to sexuality but also to one's ability to give and receive on physical and emotional levels. People whose sacral chakra flows can devote themselves to tasks and get along well with other people.

An open sacral chakra suggests not only the generation of children but also all other forms of creative action, for example, art or music.

The Solar Plexus Chakra

The solar plexus chakra is in the middle of the abdomen above the navel. Physically, it corresponds to the digestive organs such as the pancreas, stomach, liver, and gallbladder. This chakra is our power center: every person needs a natural aggressiveness in order to be able to actualize her own goals. When resistance stands in the way, force and will have to be sufficient to do away with it so you can keep going your own way.

A blockage of this chakra can, on one hand, express itself in powerlessness with aggression directed inward, but it can also manifest as an overblown desire for power that is demonstrated when the person tries to accomplish her goals with unfair methods.

The Heart Chakra

The heart chakra is situated in the middle of the chest and connects the three lower chakras with the three upper ones. It symbolizes our ability to love. A person with a developed heart chakra can take people as they are. Such people are understanding, sociable, and gladly assume social responsibility. He who listens to his heart feels the deep connections to life and not only accomplishes his own interests but also helps others accomplish their goals.

A blocked heart chakra expresses itself in lovelessness, emotionlessness, or an inner emptiness. If love is lacking or limited, it often leads to addictive behavior toward money, success, or drugs.

The Throat Chakra

The throat chakra symbolically stands for our ability to communicate openly and listen to others. On the organic level the thyroid, breathing, bronchi, vocal chords, lungs, and esophagus are all associated with the throat chakra. Thinking and feeling are unified here. A person with a harmonious throat chakra can express herself to others in an understandable way and also listen to them as well. A restriction of this chakra can manifest in shyness, stuttering, pointless chatter, or an inability to listen to others.

The Brow Chakra

The brow chakra is located between the eyes and is often called the third eye. It stands for our power to imagine, as well as for foresightedness and insight. It helps to ripen an unfinished idea into a detailed conception. People with a strongly developed third eye are sometimes able to charge their thoughts so energetically that they can be projected telepathically. If the brow chakra is blocked it can lead to nightmares, excessive anxieties, and worries, because one is not in the position to look into the future in a calm and planned manner. There is a lack of perspective.

The Crown Chakra

The crown chakra on the top of the head connects us with the spiritual world and the origin of all being. If this energy center is open we receive inspiration, have good intuition, a lot of spiritual energy, and deep insight into the interconnections of life. He who feels connected with the spiritual world fears nothing because he is a true person of knowledge. Blockages in the crown chakra can be expressed in deep loss of orientation or mental crisis. In the second half of life, a blocked crown chakra can lead to feelings of fear, uprootedness, or loneliness.

THE AURA

There are many levels of aura that surround and reflect our beings. The most important levels for working with New Homeopathy are the following:

- Physical aura, very close to the body itself
- Emotional aura, in which our feelings and moods are stored
- Mental aura, in which our mental patterns are stored
- Spiritual aura, which makes our connection to the spiritual world possible

---

CASE STUDY

Chakra Treatment

A music teacher bought a rare African stringed instrument on which three thick strings made of leather were affixed.

Every time he tried to play the instrument he immediately began to shiver and itch all over his body. He couldn't play the instrument, but still wanted to keep it. The testing of his aura resulted in a reading of grade 7 on the emotional level, and the testing of the chakras showed a blockage of the sacral chakra. Also the themes "guilt" and "regret" tested out at grade 7. During this process the man remembered a woman in Africa who had wanted to have an "affair" with him, but he rejected this at that time and obviously had stored feelings of guilt that were still present. As the optimal method of therapy we tested for a ritual of forgiveness using fire.

Two days later the music teacher reported to me that the itching had disappeared completely and he was now able to play the instrument without any symptoms.

AURA AND CHAKRA BALANCE

Aura and chakra therapy is very much a sensory work: it requires feeling yourself into things, allowing yourself into the vibrations of the patient. Since these vibrations often include unresolved emotions and old conflicts, strong emotions of grief or rage can be released during a session. Practitioners should have the training and the skill to deal with this kind of release before undertaking the work, and they should naturally be as open as possible to whatever comes along.

Aura levels and chakras can be tested by means of the tensor. Simply guide your thoughts to the relevant area or point to it with an index finger and inquire whether it is free or blocked. If an aura level or chakra tests out at anything worse than grade 5, a blockage is present. This means that the region of energy and also the corresponding organs or glands are not optimally supplied with life energy, and might sooner or later cause maladies.

Treatment of aura and chakra blockages is nicely accomplished with tones, rhythms, colors, work with revising belief patterns, or special healing rituals. Experience shows that a disturbance in the emotional aura reacts very well to tones, colors, and rituals, while a blockage in the mental aura is often better treated with the revision of belief patterns.

14

Using Tones and Rhythms

Heavenly sounds or hellish noise: since the Japanese scientist Masaru Emoto demonstrated how harmonious or disharmonious music produces beautifully structured water crystals or chaotic forms, we can begin to imagine how profoundly sound can affect us. With the help of New Homeopathy methods, tones and rhythms can be used to strengthen the life force and promote healing of all kinds.

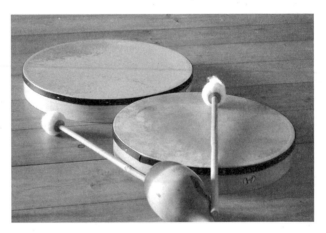

Tones and rhythms can be used
to strengthen the life force.

While sound vibrations can certainly influence the refined sensors of our chakras and auras, they can also imprint themselves on the fluid in our tissues, which makes up the greatest part of our human organism. In this way sound waves can have a health-promoting or sickness-provoking effect. With the correct "tuning music" we can rectify out-of-tune circumstances and thus support the organism in bringing itself back into harmonious tune.

COLOR AND TONE CORRESPONDENCES IN TRADITIONAL SYMBOLISM

Color	Tone	Body Reference	Emotion	Functional Principle
Red	C	Breathing	Activity, dynamism, temperament	Momentum, acceleration
Orange	D	Material exchange	Joy, liveliness, affirmation of life	Creative force, emanation
Yellow	E	Nervous system	Maturity, good cheer, change	Knowledge, expression
Green	F	Movement	Power to succeed, perseverance, relaxation, rest	Gravity, concentration
Light Blue	G	Sensory perception	Breadth, distance	Expansion, optimization
Dark Blue	A	Circulation of fluids	Satisfaction, hope, eternity	Harmony, longing
Violet	B	Regeneration	Self-centeredness, solitude, sufficiency	Imagination, reflection

There have been many scientific investigations, philosophies, methods, and classifications of music throughout history. Tones can be ascribed to planetary frequencies (Joachim-Ernst Berendt, Hans Cousto), to colors (Isaac Newton), to emotions, and to body functions. According to investigations, the unborn prefer to listen to Mozart (Alfred A. Tomatis), and our whole life is imprinted by rhythm (Rudolf Steiner), just to name a few studies selected from the wide field of music, rhythm, and colors.

METHODS OF MUSICAL THERAPY

The therapeutic use of tones or music can be effectively augmented by the methods of New Homeopathy. For example, therapists using musical bowls can use a tensor to test which bowl with which frequency should be placed on a particular part of the patient's body. We can also test how many times the bowl should be struck and how long this vibration will do any good. Thus the client will receive the individualized and optimal "dose of sound."

Healing tones or healing music can furthermore be imprinted on stones. If testing has revealed a particular healing tone, this frequency can be transferred to a stone by having the patient hold the stone in his right hand (instead of the glass of water as is done in a water transfer) while the therapist strikes the instrument. This healing tone or music does not have anything to do with the normal theory of harmonies—perhaps the tones will not sound all that beautiful to our ears—but nevertheless this vibration will provide a positive healing impulse to the patient. A healing stone, charged in this way, can then be carried every day, for as long as the testing recommended it. In this manner it is also possible to transfer healing mantras.

A further variant is aura clearing with rhythms and tones. This combination of New Homeopathy with elements of shamanism was devised by Erich Körbler. It is best to use this method in a group of people: The one receiving treatment stands in the middle, the other participants stand in a surrounding circle. Participants take musical instruments, such as rattles, cymbals, and bells, in their hands and then let these musical instruments resound in the aura of the patient. Even loud and unrhythmic sequences of sounds can result in a healing impulse. In shamanism it is just this "non-rhythm" that induces the trance, in that non-rhythmic drumming puts the brain into the so-called Alpha-state, a virtually primeval condition.

This aura cleansing is continued by the participants until the tensor of the group leader indicates that the time of this individual dose of sound has been concluded. The treatment has a very thorough, purifying, and clarifying effect.

CASE STUDY

Learning Difficulties

Alina, about eight years old, was slower than her fellow pupils in understanding things. For this reason she had problems with her teacher and received poor grades at school. Alina's mother said that during homework assignments, Alina had trouble grasping new concepts and ideas. Even when she did get it, her understanding often did not last, and her mother had to re-explain the assignments several times. Alina's mother thought this could have something to do with the medicines she took when she was pregnant with Alina.

We worked with a healing tone imprinted on a stone and tested out two water transfers, which contained two different concepts around the themes of learning, understanding, and comprehension. Testing also revealed a hand injury that Alina had as a small child, as well as the emotions attached to this. In conclusion we cleared the medicines taken during pregnancy. Alina placed the stone under her pillow for sixteen nights and performed the first water transfer. She took a break for a week and then did the second water transfer. At first her mother did not notice any improvement, but Alina got an "A" on her next math test and two days later brought home an "A" on her German test! Alina's classmates came up to her to congratulate her. The whole family beamed and was happy for her success—and I was too!

15

Using Color and Light

The cells of all living beings radiate electromagnetic vibrations. Besides visible light, we radiate vibrations of light in all directions. Through so-called *biophotons*, cells communicate with one another. Colors are visible frequencies of light that can support the powers of self-healing just as well as symbols and tones.

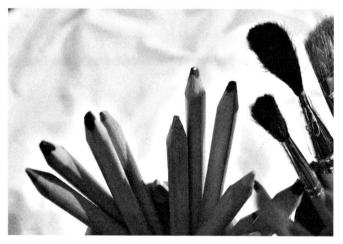

Colors can support the powers of self-healing.

In a multi-year study a team of Russian researchers succeeded in proving that there are circulatory channels for light in the human body that correspond precisely to the meridians. With the help of colored light, information can be sent into the body through acupuncture points or across large bodily zones, thereby equalizing disharmonies on an energetic level.

COLOR THERAPY

Use the tensor to determine which color is needed by having the patient look at color samples and seeing how the tensor responds. A grade 1 reading tells you that you have found a good therapeutic color.

After testing for the optimal color you can undertake an illumination with a colored lamp or shine light on individual acupuncture points with a small pocket light equipped with special changeable color filters. By drawing symbols with colored markers or writing on colored paper, you can combine symbols with the proper color to optimize their effects.

THE ENERGETIC EFFECTS OF COLORS

Various color theories associate body organ functions with specific colors. You can use the list below to determine what colors your patient is likely to benefit from, although you should always use the tensor to confirm.

- **Red** increases activity, combats fatigue, encourages blood circulation, and stimulates the metabolism. The color red supports the power of the sexual organs. Red corresponds to the root chakra.
- **Orange** works positively on the vital powers of the kidneys, supports lung tissue, works against congestion, and loosens

emotional tensions. It is an inspiring and stimulating color. Orange helps depressed or lethargic people; it is the color of joy and openness. Orange corresponds to the sacral chakra.

- **Yellow** has a positive influence on the nerves and works to promote the function of the stomach, intestines, liver, spleen, and bladder. Yellow works very well against depression. Yellow is also the color of creativity, joy, and curiosity. It corresponds to the solar plexus chakra.

- **Green** symbolizes harmony and is the color of balance. Being radiated with green light soothes the nervous system and the physical body. Green works well on stress, nervousness, and sleep disorders. Green corresponds to the heart chakra.

- **Blue** has an antiseptic and cooling effect. It reduces the heart rate, has an analgesic effect, hinders fever, and nourishes the nervous system. Blue is the color of self-observation and introspection. Blue corresponds to the throat chakra.

- **Indigo** is effective for nervous and spiritual disturbances and stimulates the pituitary gland. Through its high vibratory rate, indigo has a narcotic effect and a healing effect on burns. Indigo corresponds to the brow/third eye chakra.

- **Violet** stimulates the spiritual field. It has a balancing effect on depression and migraines and promotes the development of visions during meditation. A mixture of red and blue, violet unifies two opposites: life, fire, force (red) with rest, calmness, and introspection (blue). Violet corresponds to the crown chakra.

16
Transforming Belief Patterns

Unhealthy thoughts or belief patterns can work themselves out negatively in our bodies and minds. Based on the methods of O. Carl Simonton, our symbols can be used to rewrite unhealthy belief patterns in order to bring the biochemistry of the emotions back into harmony.

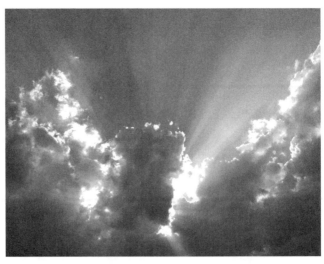

*Unhealthy belief patterns must be rewritten to bring
the body and mind back into harmony.*

We all know the phenomena we call the self-fulfilling prophecy: what we believe to be true often shapes—and limits—our experience of reality. In the psychological fight against disease, a positive basic attitude and a firm conviction that one will be healed can be a key to success. Negative convictions, on the other hand, (like "No one can help me") can have the opposite effect.

In response to these ideas the American cancer researcher O. Carl Simonton developed a special therapy for cancer sufferers. With great success Simonton called upon his cancer patients to conduct a war against the degenerate cancer cells. In guided meditations the immune system was encouraged to engage in this war. Patients were to imagine the cancer cells being targeted by the applied cancer therapy; healthy cells were employed to help in the destruction of the cancer cells. The results of this visualization were amazing. With many patients the treatment was so effective that the cancer had disappeared within a few months. The healings went well and extremely quickly, and the psychically strengthened and healthy cells were more resistant to the side effects of radiation and chemotherapy as well.

RESETTING BELIEF PATTERNS

Convictions and belief patterns steer our behavior and perception and decisively influence our lives and our health. Many people carry around belief patterns they have been collecting since childhood (from parents, teachers, etc.) and storing in their subconscious minds. With New Homeopathy we do a sort of "reset"—we erase information that is detrimental to our development and replace it with a beneficial thought-form.

In practice it is done like this:

1. Fold a sheet of paper in the middle. On the left side write the belief pattern that is to be erased; then use the tensor to determine the appropriate sign of reversal for it.

2. Draw the code over the belief pattern.

3. On the right side of the sheet the therapist and the patient work out what the positive form of this belief pattern would be, creating a carefully worded positive affirmation. See the table below for examples of effective and appropriate affirmations. The affirmation is written on the right side of the sheet, and the Ypsilon (Y) is drawn on top of it.

4. Then transfer of all this information into water, testing as described in chapter 10 as to how long the water should be drunk.

CREATING POSITIVE AFFIRMATIONS

Negative Belief Pattern	Positive Belief Pattern
I cannot do this.	I am open to new possibilities that are being offered in my life. Through these I can experience much that is new. This enriches my life and gives me joy and satisfaction.
I am not worthy, I don't deserve it.	Every person is a creation of God. Health, prosperity, love, and joy correspond to my divine nature.
I have to work hard for everything.	The quality of playful lightheartedness may now enter my life more and more. My work is more fun and joyous and everything is effortless for me.

CASE STUDY

Bedwetting at Seven Years of Age

Corina, seven years old, was still wetting the bed at night. For this reason her mother brought her to my office. First I conducted the energy balance. Then we worked on the theme "Bedwetting at Night" with the appropriate bar code. I tested for the dosage and duration of treatment, and we transferred the vibration onto blank homeopathic pellets.

A few weeks later Corina's mother called me. She reported that all was well as long as Corina had been taking the pellets, but now that they were gone, she was wetting the bed again.

At the next appointment I redid the energy balance and painted the points that had been tested out onto Corina's body. Then we worked on her problem of bedwetting with the psycho-meridian. The fourth year of life was indicated; from the emotion mandala (a special chart where emotions are related to the five elements of traditional Chinese medicine) the concepts "desperate," "there is no place for me here," and "superfluous" tested out. All of these words were written with the name of the patient and the problem on a piece of paper, and the corresponding sign was marked on it. The duration and dose of treatment were precisely tested for, and this time Corina transferred the vibration into water. Corina also painted a picture for me, which we wrapped and marked with different bar codes that had been tested out. Corina hung the picture up in her room for the time period indicated by testing.

At the next visit "three years old," "January," and "stressed" tested positive, so we worked on these themes accordingly. It turned out that when Corina was three her brother suffered a serious accident. He came home in a disabled state, confined to a wheelchair and needing constant care. In a family with four children and their own business to run, this was certainly a difficult situation that could not leave the other family members unaffected. About three months later I spoke on the phone again with the mother: Corina was doing well, the problem of bedwetting had been completely resolved.

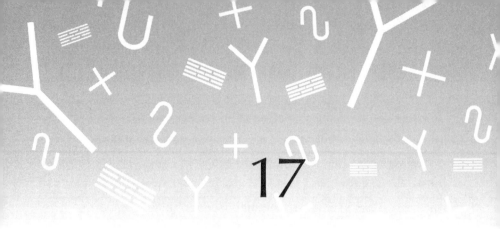

17

Working with Animals and Plants

The gentle testing and balancing methods of New Homeopathy can easily be applied to any living organism, including animals and plants. Plants plagued with parasites, for instance, can be helped by

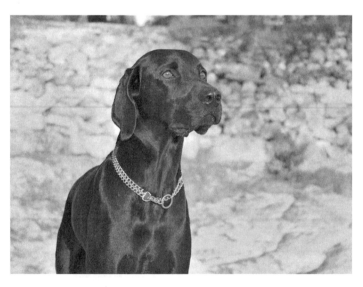

We can apply our knowledge of testing and balancing with symbols to our animal companions.

informing the water used to nourish them, while animals can be cured of a variety of maladies with water transfers as well as symbols painted directly on their bodies. Even polluted water or low-yielding fields, for example, have shown highly promising responses to this medicine. Be creative and do your own experiments: you will be amazed what will work!

WORKING WITH ANIMALS

Diseases and behavioral problems in dogs, cats, horses, and other animals can arise from bad nutrition, stress, or other dissonance in the energy field. As with humans an animal's physical symptoms can be linked to a conflict from years before, or to a hidden allergy, or to problems with feeding, among other things. We should also not forget that animals sometimes express their owner's imbalances: their symptoms often disappear once the owner is able to resolve his own conflicts. In this sense, too, animals are our good friends and helpers. They point out our own issues to us.

With animals, just like with humans, the combination of symbols works with the meridians and the energy system of the body. Functional disturbances in the organism will impair the free flow of energy through the meridian system.

HOW TO TEST ANIMALS

With the tensor you can test the overall condition of an animal or inquire about a specific organ or system. If the animal lives with other animals—in a stall or a cage, for example—test its tolerances to the neighbors, and perhaps you will end up improving conditions for several animals at the same time.

For allergic reactions or other intolerances, use the symbol of reversal, just as you might do with a person. When a horse can no longer tolerate his hay, for example, write the word "hay" and the symbol indicated by the energy circle onto a piece of paper. Then transfer this information into water or into an apple or carrot that the animal will eat. You can also paint the healing signs directly on the animal, right on the inflamed location. Always ask about how long the symbol should remain on that location.

When working with animals don't forget to inquire about geopathic pollution, such as water veins, cross-points, and other negative influences, because animals often stand or sleep in bad locations. (Please note that there are also lovers of radiation—such as cats or snakes—who adore such places. Don't drive your cat away from its favorite spot!)

A healing impulse can be generated from many things—homeopathic medicines, light, sound, healing symbols, etc. Animals especially like to take in light, colors, and sounds. Cows, for example, love the color pink and classical music, and they will produce more milk when exposed to them. So whether you are working with joints, muscles, inflammations, respiratory disorders, or behavioral problems, an experiment with color and music is always worth a try.

ANIMAL CASE STUDIES

Any animal can be treated with the New Homeopathy methods. What follows are a few examples of work with horses and with pet rabbits and guinea pigs.

CASE STUDIES: HORSES

Choke

Gordon, a four-year-old gelding, had all the typical symptoms of choke: his neck cramped, he choked, trembled, and his flanks cramped. While the veterinarian was on his way over, I tested for disturbances with the tensor.

Severe disturbances were indicated in the middle of the neck and in the flanks. I painted these areas with the appropriate bar codes, and after only about five seconds the congestion began to resolve. Feed-mush ran out of Gordon's mouth and nose, and after a few minutes he calmed down and stood in his stall—a little stressed, but quiet. When the veterinarian came he could not find any sign of the problem. The tensor indicated that the signs were to be worn for just a day. The next morning the signs were removed and Gordon showed no further indications of sickness.

Zeno

We were called to see Zeno, a fourteen-year-old stallion, who had not moved for several days. The veterinarian could find no outward indication of an injury and guessed some sort of poisoning but could not make any improvement in the symptoms. When we arrived we found the stallion standing in his stall with a hanging head, dim eyes, and hanging ears. He was sweating and he did not move. We used the tensor for an energy balance and discovered disturbances in the area of the heart, pericardium, and lungs.

During the painting of the correct bar codes on the disturbed meridian points, the horse changed visibly. After just a few minutes a gleam came to his eyes, he perked up his ears again, shook himself, and drank some water. The stallion began to walk on his own after about five minutes. With the tensor we discovered an inflammation of the tendon along his fibula and imprinted the appropriate healing information on an apple, which Zeno ate immediately. The bar codes were to remain on the horse for six days, and the apples containing the healing information were to be eaten for several days. After the conclusion of the treatment, Zeno once more demonstrated "stallion-like behavior": he moved around in his stall and greeted his neighbors in their stalls with neighing.

Inflamed Upper Eyelid

The mare, City Sue, twenty-one years old, had an inflamed upper eyelid. After testing with the tensor we gave her an information apple, which she ate that evening. By the next day the inflammation had disappeared and the eye was watering just a little bit. This disturbance disappeared completely after two days.

Severe Eczema

The twenty-four-year-old mare, Fru Fru, suffered from severe eczema. She had created a wound on her belly by scratching and biting herself and presented large bloody patches on the insides of her legs. We used the tensor to inquire about allergies and learned that Fru Fru was allergic to grass. The mare ate an informed apple each day over several weeks, and her skin began to heal. After a short span of time she had some minor itching, but no longer wounded herself by biting and scratching.

Skin Problems/Poor Hair Growth

Randalf, a three-year-old gelding, suffered from skin problems and poor hair growth. Despite being fed normally he was too thin and his ribs showed.

We performed an energy balance and immediately treated

each of the disturbed meridians with the corresponding bar codes, which were to remain on the skin for ten days. During this time Randalf began to gain weight and his hair began to grow in. After only about four weeks Randalf had his full coat of hair back.

CASE STUDIES: RABBITS AND GUINEA PIGS

Kidney Failure

The owner took her dwarf rabbit to the veterinarian because it just apathetically sat in its cage with its ears hanging down. The diagnosis was kidney failure. The veterinarian gave the rabbit only two or three days to live or alternatively advised the owner to put the rabbit to sleep.

I dowsed the kidneys and received an Ypsilon as the corresponding bar code. Since the diagnosis was so dire and destructive, I painted a 10-cm Ypsilon with a very wide black marker on both sides of the rabbit. The next day the rabbit was still alive and appeared exhausted but better. After three or four days there was a marked improvement, and at the last re-examination—after twelve days—there was nothing to be seen of the disease.

Guinea Pig with a Straw Allergy

I was called to see a guinea pig that constantly sneezed and had red eyes. The animal lived in the same cage with another guinea pig, who was completely healthy. According to tests with the tensor, the guinea pig had an intolerance to the straw in its cage. The straw was switched out for sawdust, and the little patient was treated with an information transfer ("straw allergy" with the corresponding bar code).

After one day the sneezing was gone, and the animal's general condition was good.

WORKING WITH PLANTS

In closing, here is an example of treating a plant with the methods of New Homeopathy.

CASE STUDY

Treating an Oleander Plant

Since its purchase six years earlier, the oleander had never bloomed. It was always sickly and grew only slightly.

Inquiring with the tensor about the soil as well as the branches resulted in a grade 8. The oleander was removed from its pot, washed, and repotted with new soil. The branches were pruned by one-third. Now the roots as well as the leaves tested at grade 7.

With the help of a book on plants I tested some possible ailments and got a strong response in connection with red spider mites. Since the oleander was supposed to be dormant for the winter, I could not water it anymore, which ruled out a water transfer. Instead, I wrote the reversal information—"red spider mites" along with the correct bar code—on an orange-colored piece of paper and transmitted it to the soil and the sap in the branches. The orange piece of paper remained between the branches for the three months that the testing had indicated.

In the spring I tested the oleander with the question "Okay?" Afterward I tested the plant over a month-long period and came up with a bar code of a weaker level; this time the treatment was conducted via water transfer, since the winter dormant period was over. The new leaves are healthy and the oleander is now free of spider mites. As a stabilizer there was an additional week of water transfer with an Ypsilon.

Resources

Because the practices of New Homeopathy are so new to the United States, we recommend that you contact the authors through their German websites for more information.

PETRA NEUMAYER

By googling "skripthaus" and clicking on "Translate this page," you can read Petra's website www.skripthaus.com in English.

ROSWITHA STARK

By googling "heilpraxis-stark" and clicking on "Translate this page," you can read Roswitha's website www.heilpraxis-stark.de in English.

Reading the translated page for www.medizin-zum-aufmalen.de/veranstaltungen.html will provide further information about the authors and the workshops they teach. The site www.heilzeichen-shop.com sells useful products for the practice of New Homeopathy.

Index

Page numbers in *italics* indicate illustrations.

BOOKS OF RELATED INTEREST

Vibrational Medicine
The #1 Handbook of Subtle-Energy Therapies
by Richard Gerber, M.D.

Five Point Touch Therapy
Acupressure for the Emotional Body
by Pierre-Noël Delatte, M.D.

The Subtle Energy Body
The Complete Guide
by Maureen Lockhart, Ph.D.

The Complete Book of Traditional Reiki
Practical Methods for Personal and Planetary Healing
by Amy Z. Rowland

Bioharmonic Self-Massage
How to Harmonize Your Mental, Emotional, and Physical Energies
by Yves Bligny

The Encyclopedia of Healing Points
The Home Guide to Acupoint Treatment
by Roger Dalet, M.D.

Acupressure Taping
The Practice of Acutaping for Chronic Pain and Injuries
by Hans-Ulrich Hecker, M.D., and Kay Liebchen, M.D.

Shamanism for the Age of Science
Awakening the Energy Body
by Kenneth Smith

INNER TRADITIONS • BEAR & COMPANY
P.O. Box 388
Rochester, VT 05767
1-800-246-8648
www.InnerTraditions.com

Or contact your local bookseller

Morphic
Fields
9

SYMBOLS
15-Healing

Viberations
31-32 (1 = 9 = (≤)9)
          same